AF364246

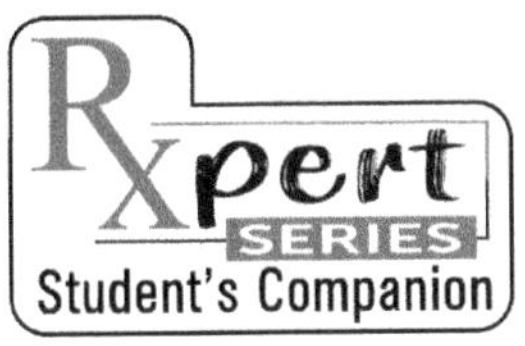

Concise

Pharmacognosy

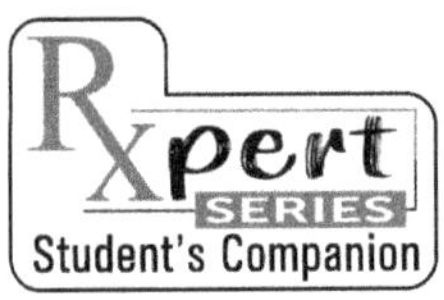

Concise
Pharmacognosy

Dr. Raveesha Peeriga

Professor & Head
Department of Pharmacognosy,
V. V. Institute of Pharmaceutical Sciences,
Gudlavalleru, Andhra Pradesh.

Dr. Lakshmana Rao Atmakuri

Principal & Professor

V. V. Institute of Pharmaceutical Sciences,
Gudlavalleru, Andhra Pradesh.

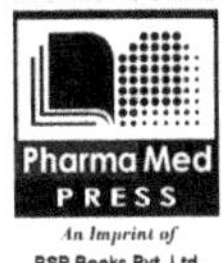

PharmaMed Press

An imprint of BSP Books Pvt. Ltd

4-4-309/316, Giriraj Lane,
Sultan Bazar, Hyderabad - 500 095.

Concise **Pharmacognosy**

by **Dr. Raveesha Peeriga and Dr. Lakshmana Rao Atmakuri**

Published by:

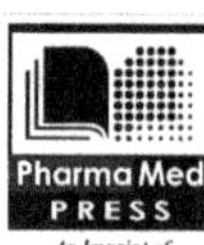

PharmaMed Press

An imprint of BSP Books Pvt. Ltd.

4-4-309/316, Giriraj Lane, Sultan Bazar, Hyderabad - 500 095.
Phone: 040-23445688; Fax: 91+40-23445611
e-mail: info@pharmamedpress.com
www.pharmamedpress.com/pharmamedpress.net

ISBN: 978-93-95039-90-1 (Hardback)

Preface

The first edition of the textbook Concise Pharmacognosy is based on curriculum of Diploma in Pharmacy. It represents the key points on historical aspects of development of Pharmacognosy and its importance. It explains about the classification of crude drugs in systemic manner. It explores about the quality control of herbal drugs. It briefly gives an outline on secondary metabolites.

The book also discusses about some of the crude drugs categorized under different therapeutics. It gives the information on natural fibres in surgical dressings and explains the importance of various traditional system of Medicine. It also represents about the importance of nutraceuticals and cosmetics of natural origin. It explores about investigation of crude drugs phytochemically.

The current book is written for ease understanding and memorizing the Pharmacognosy subject at Diploma level. I believe this book brings the educational need of Diploma students. We thank to the Almighty. We express our immense pleasure to the family members for their support. I am grateful and my sincere thanks to Dr. A. Lakshmana Rao for the guidance to complete this book. We are thankful to the Management of V. V. Institute of Pharmaceutical Sciences.

We thank the publisher, BS Publications and the staff members for their cooperation to bring forth this book.

Dr. Raveesha Peeriga
Dr. Lakshmana Rao Atmakuri

Contents

Chapter – 1

Introduction to Pharmacognosy

Chapter – 2

Classification of Crude Drugs

Chapter – 3

Quality Control of Crude Drugs

Chapter – 4

Secondary Metabolites

Chapter – 5

Crude Drugs

Chapter – 6

Plant Fibres

Chapter – 7

Traditional System of Medicine

Chapter – 8

Role of Medicinal and Aromatic Plants in National Economy and their Export Potential

Introduction to Pharmacognosy

Definition

- The words "pharmacognosy" and "gnosis" are Greek words that mean "drug" and "knowledge," respectively. J.A. Schmidt (1811) and C.A. Seydler (1815), respectively, initially used it and used it to describe the area of medicine or product that works with crude pharmaceuticals.

- J.A. Schmidt (1759–1809), an Austrian physician, first used the term "pharmacognosy" in his handwritten manuscript, "Lehrbuch der Materia Medica."

- Pharmacognosy today includes research on the physical, chemical, biochemical, and biological characteristics of medications, drug substances, or potential drugs or drug substances derived from natural sources.

- Pharmacognosy, according to the American Society of Pharmacognosy, is the study of the physical, chemical, biochemical, and biological characteristics of drugs, drug substances, or potential drugs or drug substances derived from natural sources, as well as the pursuit of novel drugs derived from these sources.

History of Pharmacognosy

- The interdependence of the biotic and abiotic components of nature makes it a prime example of the remarkable phenomenon of symbiosis.

- There is a complete supply of natural cures for every ailment known to man.

- Because of man's natural curiosity, the knowledge of medications has collected over thousands of years, and as a result, we now have numerous efficient ways to ensure health care.

- The majority of medications utilised in the past came from plants, which served as man's sole chemist for a long time. As long as humans have existed, herbal remedies have a long history.

- The ancient writings, some of which date back thousands of years, indicated that plants were utilised medicinally in China, India, Egypt, and Greece long before the Christian era.

- The Papyrus Ebers scroll, which is around 60 feet long and a foot wide and dates to the sixteenth century before Christ, is one of the most well-known relics still in existence. More than 800 equations and 700 distinct medications make up the majority of the document's material.

- Crude extracts were employed for the majority of the medicinally effective compounds discovered in the nineteenth and twentieth centuries. Since 5000 B.C., numerous medicinal herbs have been used in China.

- Pen-t'sao, a text created by Emperor Shen Nung circa 3000 B.C., is the oldest herbal known to exist. There are 365 medications in it, one for every day of the year. Indians also laboriously examined and categorised the herbs they encountered into categories known as Gunas.

- According to Charaka, fifty groups of ten plants would be sufficient to meet the needs of a typical doctor. Similar to this, Sushrutha categorised 760 herbs into 7 different groups based on some of their shared characteristics. A large portion of the Indian population even today depends on the Indian System of Medicine - Ayurveda, 'An ancient science of life'. The well known treatises on Ayurveda are Charaka Samhita and Sushrutha Samhita.

- It is well known that the first pharmacist, Galen, kept opium and other painkillers in his apothecary.

- Following that, several daring attempts were undertaken to create mineral salts that may have had the potential to be used as all-purpose therapeutic agents by chemical entrepreneurs like Paracelsus (1493–1541).

- Le'mery reported on the significance of the extraction process and alcohol as an extractant (1645-1715).

- Based on ten years of research, William Withering provided an explanation of some of the medicinal qualities of foxglove leaves in 1785.

- The crude medicines were produced using the percolation procedure. In 1788, the alkaloidal drug calumba was made legal.

- Derosne, a French pharmacist, separated narcotine from opium in 1803.

- Morphine was first isolated from opium by Sertuerner in 1806, and its use in treating pain was later recognised.

- Strychnine 11817, emetine 11817, brucine (1819), piperine (1819), quinine (1820), and colchicine (1820) were isolated over the following several years.

- Strychnine was initially isolated from Ignatius beans and then from Nux vomica seeds by the French pharmacologist Pelletier.

- Stan and Otto created a new method of alkaloid extraction in 1852.

- Podophyllotoxin (Kuersten, 18911), cocaine (Neumann, 1860), ouabain (Hardy and Gallows, 1877), pilocarpine (Gerrard and Hardy,1875), ephedrine (Nagai, 1887), and nicotine were all isolated from tobacco leaves during this time period.

- The key discoveries of the 20th century were the isolation of ergometrine, digoxin, reserpine, theophylline, and quinidine.

- In the nineteenth century, the field of study today known as "Pharmacognosy" was known as Materia Medica.

- In the title of his book Analecta Pharmacognostica, German scientist Seydler first used the term "pharmacognosy" in 1815 while researching sarsaparilla.

- The name "pharmacognosy" comes from the Greek words "pharmakon" (drug) and "gignosco" (to acquire the knowledge of).

- Pharmacognosy is a subfield of bioscience that focuses on the analysis of primary or crude pharmaceuticals derived from plant, animal, and mineral sources. It entails knowledge of the history, distribution, cultivation, collection, processing for market and preservation, the study of sensory, physical, chemical, and structural characteristics, and the uses of crude drugs. To put it briefly, it is an objective study of crude drugs from natural sources treated scientifically.

- Swedish systematist Linnaeus (1707–1778), noted for classifying plants, developed the binomial system of plant naming, which is being used today.

- Engler and Prandtl, A.W. Eichler, Bentham and Hooker (1862–1863), and others furthered plant classification (1887-1898).

- G. Mendel's significant findings regarding plant hybrids were published in 1865. The invention of the microscope as a crucial analytical tool was a turning point in botanical research, especially because various processes, such as preparatory cleaning, mounting, and staining, were developed.

- Berg released the initial drug anatomical atlas in 1865. Voehl, Tschirch, and others described the anatomical characteristics of a number of powdered medications later in the century, which proved to be very important, especially at a time when adulteration in both drugs and food products was prevalent. Greenish and Collin created "An Anatomical Atlas of Powdered Vegetable Drugs" in 1904.

- In a nutshell, pharmacognosy serves as a vital link between the basic and pharmaceutical sciences. An essential link between the Ayurvedic and allopathic medical systems is pharmacognosy. It offers a mechanism for dispensing, formulating, and manufacturing crude pharmaceuticals using active ingredients drawn from natural sources in dose forms recognised by the allopathic medical system.

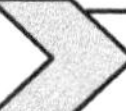 ## Development of Pharmacognosy to the Current Century

- The history of pharmacognosy development is the development of the use of plants and other natural resources for therapeutic reasons.

- The history of herbalism and the history of food are intertwined because humans have traditionally employed a variety of herbs and spices to season food and ward against infections that cause food-borne illness.

- Through observation, accidental discovery, trial-and-error guesswork, curiosity, and the pursuit of sustenance, among other methods, the ancient people studied the medical characteristics of plants and developed rudimentary medications

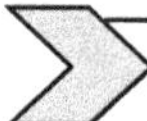 ## Trial-and-error Guesswork

- Trial-and-error guesswork refers to the practise of attempting something and then tossing it aside until it is successful. Ancient people could distinguish between useful and dangerous plants because to this technique.

- When people were nomads who subsisted on wild animal hunting and plant gathering, they employed this clumsy and time taking process for identification of herbs. Plants were employed for healing by ancient people who were guided by instinct, taste, experience, and knowledge. • In the recent years, a number of novel techniques, computer-based technology, and bio mathematical models have replaced the ineffective age-old trial-and-error guesswork method of drug discovery. They dug, dried, chewed, pounded, rubbed, and brewed many of the plants surrounding them and attempted to discover herbal effects through trial-and-error guesswork.

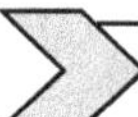 ## While Searching for Food

- Humans first discovered many of the herbs and spices they use today when looking for plants to utilise as food. Later, they learned that many plants also have medicinal properties.

- For thousands of years, people from all cultures have utilised spices and herbs to improve the flavour and scent of food.

- Early societies also valued the use of spices and herbs for both their culinary and medicinal purposes.

- Numerous spices, herbs, and their components have been shown to possess antibacterial properties in scientific studies since the late nineteenth century.

- The ancient people used the plants and spices they had acquired over time, learning about their virtues as they went along.

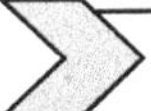

Signature of Nature

- The anatomical structures of many naturally occurring plants or their parts superficially resemble those of humans. While looking for and choosing plants for therapeutic usage, the ancient people may have placed stress on specific "signatures" likeness between plant and sick organ.

- These blatant structural resemblances served as the selection standard for therapeutic application. Ancient trademark plants include horsetail, gingko, ginseng, and others. In the past, numerous societies independently established their own versions of this concept. Later, it gained notoriety as the "Doctrine of Signature."

- The Doctrine of Signatures has likely been around for as long as there have been humans who study plants.

- The configuration and structure of a plant influenced early man to use it in the treatment of various diseases, for example, horsetail mimics cartilage and was believed to support the connective tissue, leaves; the cross section of the Ginkgo biloba fruit resembles a brain and today, Ginkgo is used for memory loss; and ginseng root resembles the human body and has been used for thousands of years as a tonic for the entire body.

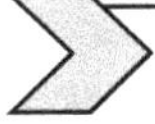

Animal's Instinctive Discrimination between Toxic and Palatable Plants

- Animals can automatically distinguish between poisonous and appetising plants to survive in an unpredict environment. Ancient people observed animal behaviour closely and discovered that sick animals used some herbs that they ordinarily avoid.

- Ancient people were able to select medicinally beneficial plants by carefully and intimately observing the instinctual behaviour of animals.

- Many other animals, such as birds, bees, cats, dogs, elephants, elk, lizards, and different carnivores, are also known to consume medicinal plants for self-medication, according to growing scientific evidence. Examples include chimpanzees eating Aspilia shrub and pith of Veronia plant to remove parasitic worms from the intestinal lining (zoopharmacognosy).

- This technique is still used by scientists today to separate active components from therapeutic plants.

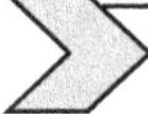

Accidental Discovery/Fortuitous Accidents

- Plants have been used as medicines since antiquity, and some of these plants may have been unintentionally found (unexpected discoveries by accident).

- By mistake, a South American discovered the antimalarial medication quinine from Cinchona bark (also known as quina-quina by native people), and the antibiotic penicillin from Pencillium mould.

- The unintentional findings are known as drug serendipity (finding of one thing while looking for something else).

- There are several instances of therapeutic plants and their components being discovered by accident.

- Cannabis has been used medicinally for at least 5000 years, although Cannabis sativa's medicinal uses were only discovered by accident. Cannabis is a potent medical plant well-known for its hallucinogenic qualities.

- Serendipitous or accidental discoveries have led to some of the most significant medical advancements of our time, including the smallpox vaccine, insulin and its application in the treatment of diabetes, X-rays, and Viagra.

- People of all times have used plants as their primary source of food, shelter, and medicine.

- Since 5000 BC, medicinal herbs have been used in China. The oldest pharmacopoeia known to exist is thought to be the Chinese "Pen T'sao," which was composed by Shen nung around 3000 BC. It listed 365 medications.

- The "Pen T'sao Jing Ji Zhu", composed by Tao Hong Jing (456–536 AD), contains 730 herbs in six categories, including minerals, grasses and trees, insects and animals, fruits and vegetables, and grains.

- The Indian subcontinent was known among ancient civilizations as a rich source of medicinal herbs. The ancient medicine of classical antiquity known as Ayurveda (Ayur means life, veda means the study of, i.e., life, knowledge), has codified almost 8000 herbal medicines.

- Based on four Hindu Vedas (e.g., the Rig, the Sama, the Yajur, and the Atharva Vedas) that were compiled/written in ancient Sanskrit between 6000 and 4000 BC, Ayurveda underwent major development during the Vedic period. Out of them, the Atharva Veda and the Rig Veda are some of the earliest written records regarding the medical knowledge and practises that served as the foundation of the Ayurveda system. The Rig Veda is the oldest written book that has been maintained in a library.

- 67 species of medicinal plants were described in the Rig Veda, 81 in the Yajur Veda, and 290 in the Atharva Vaveda. Characteristics and applications of 1100 and 1270 species, respectively, were covered in the Charak Samhita and the Sushrut Samhita.

- The greater triad, which includes the Astanga Sangraha, the Charaka Samhita, and the Sushruta Samhita, is composed of key texts in ayurveda and was authored by Charaka, Sushruta, and Vagbhata, respectively.

- Sushruta Samhita later provided details on a large number of the plants (700), minerals (64), and animal preparations (57) utilised in Ayurveda.

- Following the construction of state hospitals for Ayurveda in various regions of the nation, Ayurveda is currently well integrated into the Indian national healthcare system.

- On papyrus, the ancient Egyptians recorded their medical practises and procedures. The use of papyrus as a writing surface dates back to antiquity. Papyrus is a thick type of paper manufactured from the pith of the papyrus plant (Cyperus papyrus).

- For centuries after Theophrastus, the first systematic treatment of the botanical world—Historia Plantarum—remains crucial for both herbalists and botanists. Greek herbalist Krateus (100 BC) wrote a text on therapeutic plants with illustrations. His impact can be seen in Dioscorides' De Materia Medica and other writings. Dioscorides, the founder of pharmacognosy, was a Roman army medical officer and pharmacognosist who investigated therapeutic plants wherever he went. In 78 AD, he released five volumes of "De Materia Medica," a work on pharmacopoeia.

- Galen's considerable study on the four basic characteristics and the humours enabled pharmacists to more accurately adjust their prescriptions for each patient's particular symptoms. The idea of Galen formed the basis of both allopathic and homeopathic systems of medicine practiced today (Sofowora 1982).

- As pharmacy and medicine developed gradually, pharmacognosy served as their foundation. Brunfels (1488–1534) grouped herbs in an alphabetical list with drawings in his initial work in botany. Bock (1498–1554) continued Brunfels' work in a more scientific manner and created the groundwork for Linnaeus by classifying plants for the first time into herbs, shrubs, and trees. He provided detailed descriptions of the plants in his herbal, creating the first example of phytography. At least 100 new plants that were not previously mentioned in the writings of Dioscorides, Pliny, and Galen were added by Fuchs (1501–1577 AD) to his herbal. A well-known herbalist of the sixteenth century, Mattioli (1500–1577 AD), included numerous herbs from the New World in his formulations.

- The 'Doctrine of Signatures' was a concept long held by herbalists before it was introduced by well-known German alchemist and herbalist Paracleus (1493–1541). The doctrine of signatures is the concept that everything was created by God with a sign (a signature), and that the sign served as a clue as to why it was made.

- The term "Pharmacognosy" was originally used by Austrian J.A. Schmidt (1759-1809) in a manuscript that was posthumously published in 1811, and it was used by German C.A. Seydler in his book in 1815 to cover medications with plant origins.

- Microscopy was first used in pharmacognosy in the nineteenth century to check the quality of unprocessed medications, and for many years, pharmacognosy was restricted to the study of crude drugs.

- The discovery of significant medications from the animal world and microbes, in particular hormones and vitamins, have become a highly important source of drugs in the twentieth century.

- Thin layer chromatography (TLC), gas chromatography (GC), high-pressure liquid chromatography (HPLC), and spectrometric approaches (MS, NMR) were developed for pharmacognostical analysis and the search for novel physiologically active chemicals in plants in the second half of the 20th century. Due to the variety of qualities that plants possess as well as their lack of harmful side effects, many alternative doctors in the twenty-first century use herbalism in modern medicine.

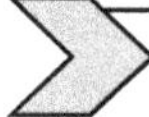

Scope of Pharmacognosy

- Early on (between the nineteenth and second part of the twentieth centuries), pharmacognosy was created as a descriptive botanical discipline. At the moment, plant-based medications are being studied and produced within the context of contemporary medicine.

- The discovery, characterization, manufacture, and standardisation of natural medicines have all benefited from pharmacognosy.

- As a result, pharmacognosy has a wide range of applications and encompasses the scientific study of medical goods such as excipients, enzymes, vitamins, antibiotics, insecticides, and allergies (e.g., coloring, flavuring, emulsifying and suspending agents, diluents etc)

- The progress of numerous science departments has benefited greatly from the pharmacognosy.

- Pharmacognosy includes plant taxonomy, plant breeding, plant pathology, and plant genetics, and by using this knowledge, one can enhance the cultivation techniques for both medicinal and aromatic plants. Pharmacognosy also gives a sound understanding of the vegetable drugs under botany and the animal drugs under zoology.

- Plant chemistry, or photochemistry, has significantly improved nowadays. This encompasses a wide range of chemicals that plants both collect and manufacture.

- A crucial contribution to the progress of physical and natural science. This has been accomplished by the development of pharmaceutical collection, processing, and storage technologies through the use of cutting-edge cultivation, purification, and identification techniques for natural pharmaceuticals. Chemical engineering and biochemistry concepts have also played a role in this.

- It establishes a crucial connection between pharmacology and medicinal chemistry; it also imparts knowledge of chemotaxonomy and biogenetic pathways for the synthesis of acute components. Pharmacognosy is crucial for the development of new medicines since crude medications are used to make galanicals or as a source of therapeutically active metabolites.

- Newly discovered plant drugs are converting into medicine as purified phytochemicals. Substances that are synthesised are ultimately created in appropriate dosage forms, sometimes using the raw drugs as intermediaries.

- To put it simply, pharmacognosy plays a key role in bridging the gaps between pharmaceuticals, basic research, and the allopathic and ayurvedic medical systems.

Pharmacognosy is the science of the active ingredients of unprocessed medications, and it can aid in dosage form manufacture, dispensing, and formulation. The full understanding of pharmacognosy will also be helpful in understanding the current industrial trend. The pharmaceutical departments, innovative medication delivery methods, and other departments can all be used as research instruments to enhance healthcare infrastructure globally.

CHAPTER 2

Classification of Crude Drugs

Many pharmacological advances nowadays are based on plant-based medical practices healing. Plant-based medicine is still used by almost four billion people worldwide to treat a variety of maladies, particularly in underdeveloped nations. The invention of novel phytotherapeutic chemicals relies heavily on using plants as crude pharmaceuticals. Plants play an ubiquitous role in treatment of diseases across all medical systems. The traditional use of plants can be traced back to prehistoric times, such as Mesopotamia, where the healing virtues of plants, as well as the time of harvest, preparation method, and therapeutic function of the plant in question, were passed down from generation to generation.

Crude medications are unaltered natural formulations of plants, animals, fungus, microbes, or minerals intended to prevent or treat illness or disease. Traditional pharmacopoeias describe the formally used crude medications in traditional medicine, with around 85 percent derived from plants and 15 percent shared in a ratio of 2:1 for minerals and animal components, respectively. The pharmacopoeia may list crude medications and categories them using various criteria, such as morphological, taxonomic, alphabetical, medicinal activity, or active compounds discovered inside them.

Broadly, plant crude pharmaceuticals can be classed according to their morphology, which might be organised or disorganised. Organized crude pharmaceuticals are preparations prepared from the full organ of the plant, where it contains a specific plant tissue, and utilized for therapy, such as leaves, roots, flowers, or seeds used to treat a specific condition.

The term 'crude drug' is generally applied to the products from plant and animal origin found in a raw material. Also the term 'crude drug' is referred in relation to the natural product that has not been advanced in value or improved in condition by any process or treatment.

Crude drugs are further classified into organized drugs and unorganized drugs based upon morphology. The main drawback of morphological classification is there is no co-relation of chemical constituents with the therapeutic actions.

In Pharmacognosy, the crude drugs are classified into:

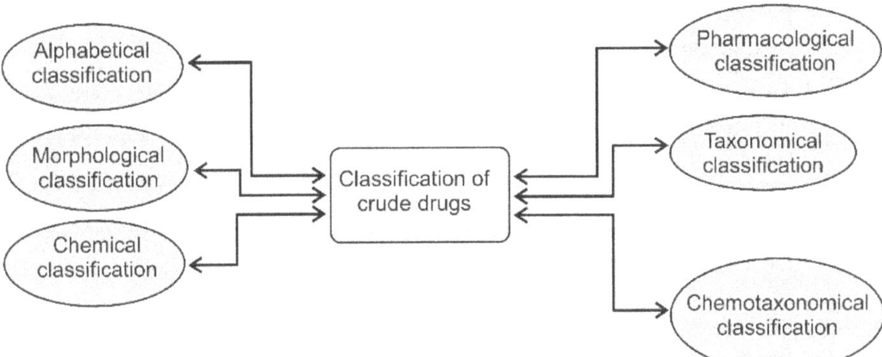

1. Alphabetical Classification:

- In this classification the drugs are arranged in alphabetical order from A to Z according to their particular language.

- In European Pharmacopoeia, the arrangement of drugs are according to their names in both 'Latin' and 'English'.

- In United States Pharmacopoeia, British Pharmacopoeia, Indian Pharmacopeia, the drugs were arranged in 'English'.

- It is a simple system as referring drugs will be at ease.

- This system of classification is a failure as the crude drugs were not categorized regarding its chemical nature, biological activity or medical uses of drugs.

Example:

Agar, Benzoin, Cinchona, Dill, Ergot, Fennel, Gentian, Hyoscyamus, Ipecac, Jalap, Kurchi, Liquorice, Myrrh, Nux-vomica, Opium, Podophyllum, Quassia, Rauwolfia, Senna, Uncaria gambier, Vasaka, Wool fat, Yellow bees wax, Zedoary.

2. Taxonomical Classification:

- In this system the crude drugs are arranged according to taxonomical features of the plant. The drugs are arranged according to their taxonomical classification - phylum, order, family, genus and species.

- This classification is purely on botanical concepts and restricted mainly to crude drugs from plant source.

- It will provide a detail description about genus and species of plants along with their taxonomical features.

- This classification has demerits as some the entire plants will not be used for therapeutic purpose but only particular parts of the plant have been processed systematically.
- This system fails because the chemical nature of active constituents and therapeutic significance of crude drugs is not considered to classify the drugs

Examples:

The taxonomical classification of Glycyrrhiza glabra

Phylum	-	Spermatophyta
Division	-	Angiospermae
Class	-	Dicotyledons
Order	-	Rosales
Family	-	Leguminosae
Genus	-	Glycyrrhiza
Species	-	Glycyrrhiza glabra

The taxonomical classification of Atropa belladonna:

Phylum	-	Spermatophyta
Division	-	Angiospermae
Class	-	Dicotyledons
Order	-	Tubiflorae
Family	-	Solanaceae
Genus	-	Atropa, Hyoscyamus, Datura
Species	-	Hyoscyamus niger, Datura stramonium, Atropa belladonna

3. Morphological Classification:

- The crude drug is categorized into organized and unorganized forms.
- The organized drugs of a plant are classified as leaves, flower, fruit, bark, root etc.,
- The unorganized drugs are dried latex, gums, extracts etc.,
- This classification is very easy in practical approach especially when the chemical nature of the drug is not known.

Example:

Seeds	-	Nux-vomica
Leaves	-	Senna
Barks	-	Cinchona

Woods	-	Quassia
Roots	-	Rauwolfia
Rhizomes	-	Turmeric
Flower	-	Saffron, Clove
Fruit	-	Coriander, Fennel
Whole plant	-	Ephedra, Ergot, Belladona
Dried latex	-	Opium, Papin
Resins	-	Balsam of Tolu, Myrrh
Gums	-	Acacia, Tragacanth, Guar gum
Dried juices	-	Aloe, Red gum
Dried extracts	-	Gelatin, Agar, Curare

4. Chemical Classification:

- Crude drugs are categorized based on chemical constituents present in the drug to which the pharmacological/therapeutic activity of drug is concerned.

- In this classification, the drugs are made easy to study if it contains a known chemical constituents.

- The different originated drugs will be under similar chemical category.

Examples:

Alkaloids	-	Datura, Vasaka, Vinca, Lobelia
Glycosides	-	Cascara, Senna, Digitalis
Tannins	-	Catechu, Myrobalan, Ashoka
Volatile oil	-	Clove, Eucalyptus, Cinnamon
Lipids	-	Castor oil, Beeswax, Arachis oil
Carbohydrates and derived products	-	Acacia, Agar, Honey, Guar gum, Tragacanth, Starch
Resins	-	Colophony, Jalap
Vitamins and hormones	-	Yeast, Shark liver oil, Insulin, Oxytocin
Proteins and enzymes	-	Gelatin, Papain, Casein, Trypsin

5. Pharmacological Classification:

- The crude drugs are grouped according to pharmacological activity (Therapeutic action) due to the presence of chief active constituents present in the crude drug.
- No morphological, taxonomical features or chemical relationships is considered.
- They can be classified on the basis of therapeutic or pharmacological effect even no ideal on chemical constituents present in it

Example:

Drugs acting on Gastro-intestinal tract:

Carminatives	-	Dill, Mentha, Cardamom
Emetics	-	Ipecac
Purgatives	-	Senna, Castor oil
Bulk laxatives	-	Agar, Banana
Anti-amoebic	-	Kurchi, Ipecac

Drugs acting on Respiratory System:

Expectorants	-	Liquorice, Ipecac, Vasaka
Antiexpectorants	-	Stramonium leaves
Antitussives	-	Opium
Bronchodilators	-	Ephedra

Drugs acting on Cardio-Vascular System:

Cardio tonics	-	Digitalis, Squill
Antihypertensives	-	Rauwolfia
Vaso-construction	-	Ergot

Drugs acting on CNS:

Central analgesics	-	Opium
CNS stimulant	-	Coffee
CNS-depressants	-	Hyoscyamus, Belladonna, Opium
Hallucinogenic	-	Cannabis, Poppy

Drugs acting as Anti-malarial:

Cinchona, Artemisia

6. Chemotaxonomical Classification:

- In this system, the crude drugs are classified based on taxonomical status and the type of chemical constituents present in it. As the type of chemical constituents are meant to the characteristic features of Phylum.

- To classify the drugs under this classification a detailed investigation of distribution of chemical compounds among different plants categorized under phylum i.e., biosynthesis related compounds in a series of related plants.

- This classification is mainly focused on chemotaxonomy of secondary metabolites possessing pharmaceutical significance viz., alkaloids, glycosides, flavonoids, etc.

CHAPTER 3

Quality Control of Crude Drugs

Adulteration is described as the partial or complete replacement of the original crude medicine with a similar-looking drug. The blended material lacks or has inferior chemical and medicinal

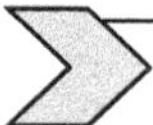

Different Methods of Adulteration of Crude Drugs

The adulteration is done deliberately or accidentally. Adulteration results due to deterioration/admixture/sophistication/substitution/Inferiority and spoilage.

- Deterioration - Impaired quality of drug.
- Admixture - Add up of one article to genuine drug due to carelessness or accidently.
- Sophistication - Intentional or deliberate type of adulteration.
- Substitution - Total different substance is replaced in place of original drug.
- Inferiority - Any substandard drug, and
- Spoilage - Due to microorganisms.

Adulteration may be due to the following reasons:

1. Adulteration Using Manufactured Substances

The original drug are replaced by the synthetic manufactured substances.

Examples

- Compressed chicory is used in case of coffee berries.
- A yellow colored Paraffin wax replaced in case of beeswax,
- Artificial invert sugar replaces honey.

2. Substitution Using Inferior Commercial Varieties

The drugs are substituted with inferior quality drugs but resembles the same in morphologically, chemically or therapeutically.

Example:

- Senna is replaced by Arabian senna.
- Ginger replaced by Japanese ginger.
- *Capsicum minimum is replaced by Capsicum annuum.*

3. Substitution Using Exhausted Drugs

The active constituents are extracted and the drugs which appears as same after extraction is reused by adding some of the coloring or flavouring agents.

Examples:

- Clove, fennel, Saffron and red rose petals, balsam of tolu etc.

4. Substitution of Superficially Similar Inferior Natural Substances

The substituent used may appear similar in morphological aspects but the drug will be entirely devoid of genuine article in their constituents or therapeutic activity.

Examples:

- Ailanthus leaves are substituted for belladona, senna, etc.
- saffron admixed with saff flower;
- clove stalks and mother cloves with cloves;
- Japan wax for beeswax

5. Adulteration Using the Vegetative Part of the Same Plant

Vegetative parts of the same genuine plant is used as an adulteration.

Examples:

- Epiphytes like mosses, liverworts grows on the bark will be retained along with the drug. e.g. cascara or cinchona.
- Excessive amount of stems in drugs like lobelia, stramonium leaves etc.

6. Addition of Toxic Materials

In this type of adulteration the materials used for adulteration would be toxic in nature.

Examples:

- Limestone pieces with asafoetida,
- Lead shot in opium,
- Amber-coloured glass pieces in colophony,
- Barium sulphate to silver grain cochineal and
- Manganese dioxide to black grain cochineal.

7. Adulteration of Powders

High rate of adulteration is associated with the powdered drugs. Powdered waste products which looks with similar colour and density is replaced in the place of genuine drug.

Examples:

- Powdered olive stones in case of gentian powder or liquorice or pepper
- Brick powder in case of bark associated crude drugs
- Red sanders wood to replace chillies

8. Addition of Synthetic Principles

Synthetic pharmaceutical principles are used for market and therapeutic value.

Examples:

- Citral is added to lemon oil whereas benzyl benzoate is added to balsam of Peru.

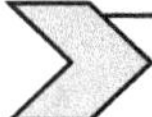 # Evaluation of Crude Drugs

- Drug evaluation establishes a drug's identity, as well as its quality and purity.
- The biochemical variations in the drug, the effects of handling and storing the drug, and adulterations and substitutes are the main causes for the requirement for examination of crude pharmaceuticals.
- Physical, chemical, biological, microscopic, and organoleptic characteristics are currently used in the evaluation of herbs.

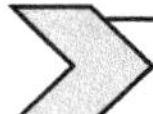 # Organoleptic Evaluation

The evaluation of medications through the sense organs is known as organolepticity.

It alludes to analytical techniques including colour, smell, taste, size, form, and unique characteristics like touch and texture.

The most basic yet humane type of study is organoleptic analysis.

Examples:

- Disc shaped - *Nux vomica* seed
- Ovoid tears acacia
- Ribbon shaped tragacanth
- Fractured structures in cinchona and Cascara bark.
- Pungent taste of Capsicum and sweet taste of liquorice.

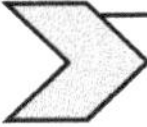 ## Microscopical Evaluation

Initial identification of herbs, the recognition of minute particles of unprocessed or powdered plants, and the detection of adulterants all require microscopic analysis.

Every plant has a unique tissue structure, which can be seen by examining how the tissues are arranged and how the cell walls and configuration are when the plant is appropriately mounted in stains, reagents, and media.

With a drop of phloroglucinol and strong hydrochloric acid, lignin stains crimson or pink.

Mucilage is dyed pink with ruthenium red, whereas starch and hemicellulose are stained blue with N/50 iodine solution.

In-depth research has been done on the distinguishing characteristics of cell walls, cell contents etc.

Example:
- Lignified trichomes in nux vomica and wavy medullary rays of cascara bark. Senna's warty trichomes.
- Sclereids and calcium oxalate crystals are present in the powder of clove stalks but not in the actual clove.

This assessment also makes use of quantitative microscopy, leaf constant determination, and microscopic linear measurements. Measurements that are linear include trichome size, fibre length and width, and starch grain size.

The cassia bark's starch grains can be distinguished from cinnamon by their diameter and the senna stalk can be found in powdered senna leaves.

Phloem fibre diameter aids in the detection of cassia in cinnamon, and vessel width aids in the detection of clove stalks in powdered cloves.

Stomatal No., Stomatal Index, Vein islet No., Vein Termination No. and palisade ratios are measurements of diameter used to identify commercial starches and to calculate leaf constants.

Stomatal number is the average number of stomata per square millimetre of a leaf's epidermis.

Stomatal index: Each stoma is counted as one epidermal cell when calculating the percentage of stomata to total epidermal cells. The formula below can be used to determine stomatal index:

$$\text{Stomatal Index(S.I.)} = S/E{+}S \times 100$$

where,

       S = number of stomata per unit area and

       E = number of epidermal cells in the same unit area.

Vein-islet Number: The number of vein islets per square millimetre of the leaf surface located halfway between the midrib and the margin is known as the vein-islet number. It serves as a defining property for a certain plant species and is used to distinguish it from related species. In 1929, Levin counted the vein-islets on various dicot leaves.

Palisade Ratio: The average number of palisade cells that lie below each epidermal cell is known as the palisade ratio.

Examples:

- Vein-islet number of Alexandrian senna is 25-29.5, whereas Indian senna is 19.5-22.5.

- Stomatal index of Alexandrian senna is 10-15, whereas that of Indian Senna is 14-20.

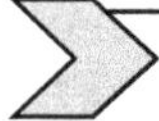 ## Stomata

The epidermis of a leaf exhibits a variety of features, such as a cuticle. trichomes, water pores, cell inclusions, stomata, etc.

A stoma is a tiny epidermal opening found on the aerial sections of plants. It has the following features. Two kidney-shaped cells with chloroplasts, known as guard cells, and a variety of subsidiary (epidermal) cells covering the guard cells make up the I central pore (ii) structure.

Gaseous exchange is the stomata's primary and most significant function, and transpiration is its secondary function.

The arrangement of stomata in dicot leaves' upper and lower epidermis varies greatly.

Types of stomata

Stomata are categorised into four kinds based on the guard cell type and subsidiary cell layout.

Depending on the shape and arrangement of subsidiary cells, dicotyledonous stomata are divided into the following kinds.

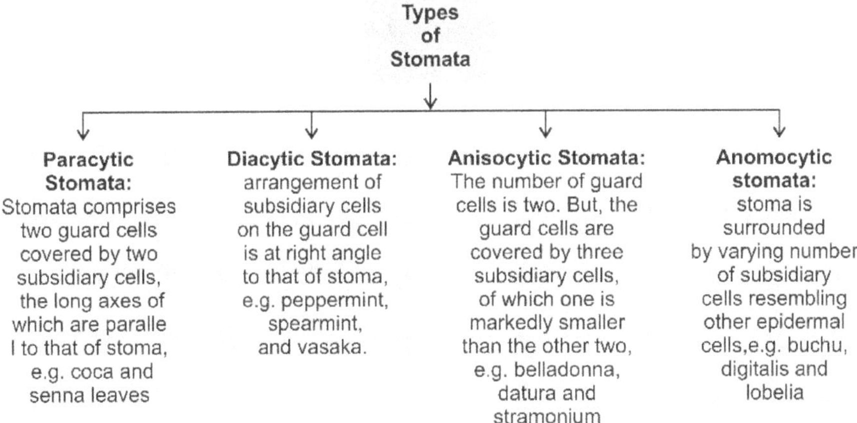

Trichomes

- These are another important diagnostic characters helpful in the identification of drugs and detection of adulterants.

- Trichomes are the tubular elongated or glandular outgrowth of the epidermal cell.

- Trichomes are also called as plant hairs.

- Trichomes consist of two parts viz., root (in the epidermis) and body (outside the epidermis).

- Trichomes are as such functionless, but sometimes, perform secretory function.

- The trichomes excrete water and at times, volatile oil as in case of peppermint.

Depending upon the structure and the number of cells present in trichomes, they are classified as given below:

1. Covering trichomes or non-globular trichomes or clothing trichomes

2. Glandular trichomes;

3. Hydathodes or special type or trichomes.

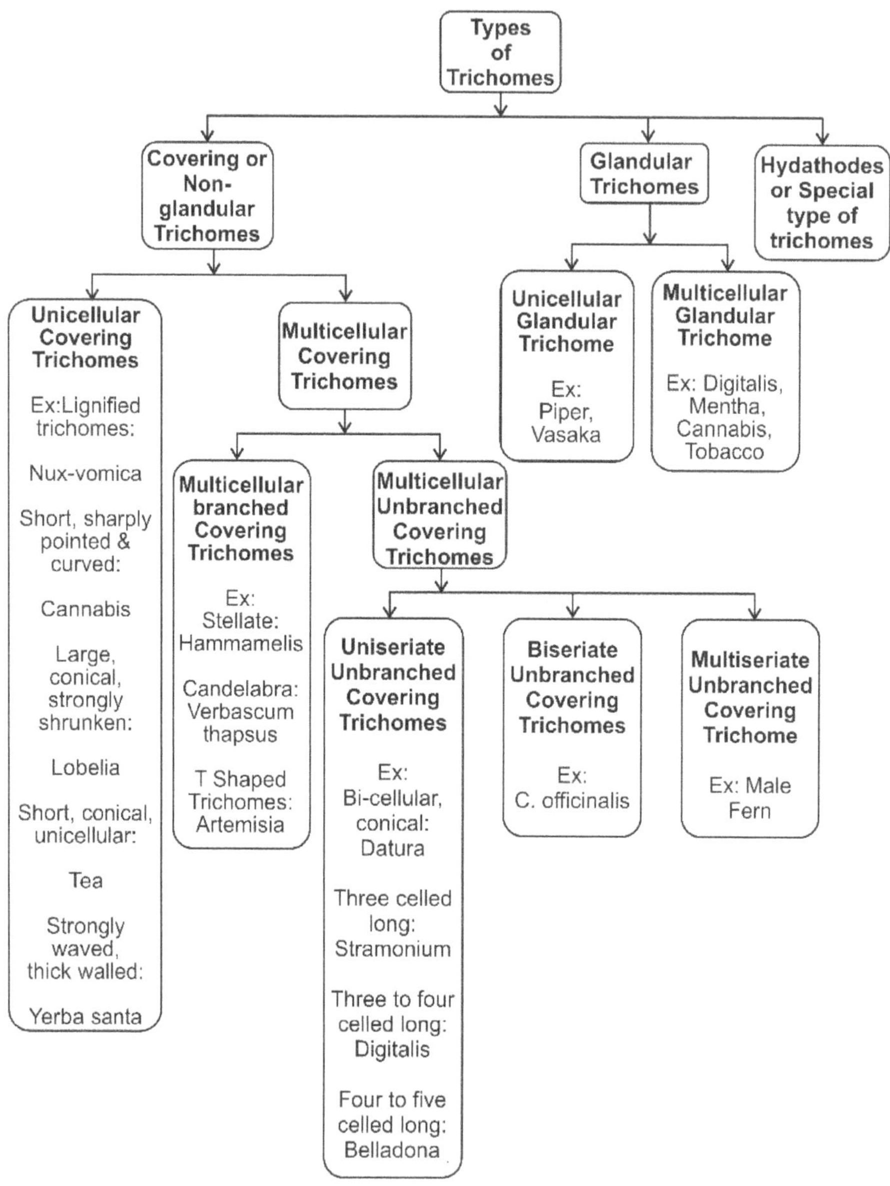

Types of Trichomes

Calcium Oxalate Crystals

The inorganic crystalline compounds by virtue of their specific shapes can be utilized for the identification of herbal drugs. Due to this reason they are known as diagnostic characters of the plant.

- Calcium oxalate is a dimorphic salt of which both the types occur in the plant body. The crystals are either monoclinic or tetragonal in shape.

- There are six forms of calcium oxalate crystals in plants as follows.

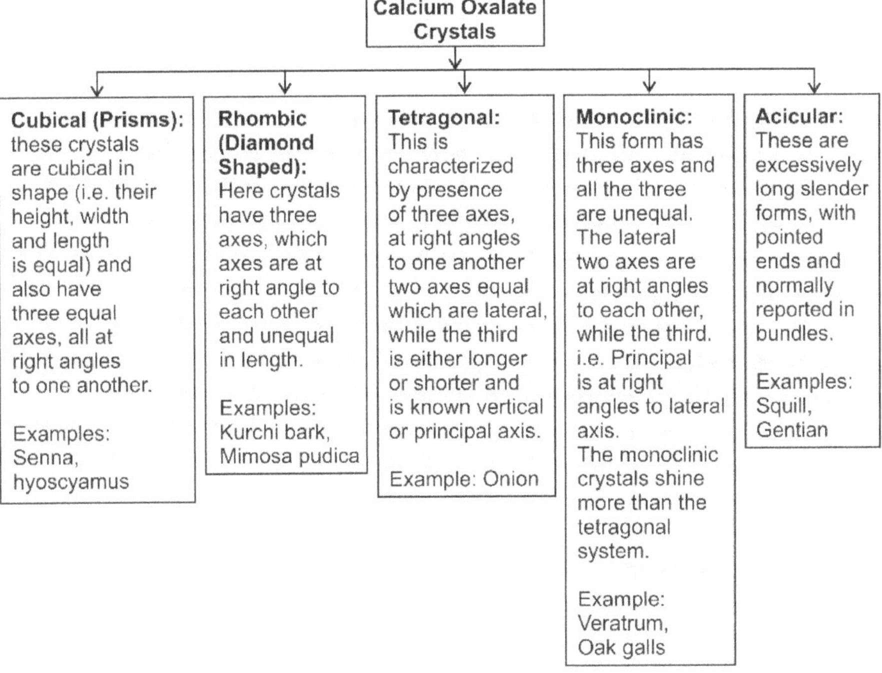

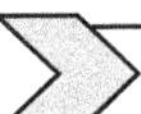 **Types of Calcium Oxalate Crystals**

Quantitative Microscopy (Lycopodium Spore Method)

- When chemical and physical approaches cannot be used to identify crude drugs, this vital technique is used. This allows one to use the Lycopodium spore method to determine the proportions of the compounds present using a microscope.

- This method is typically used to evaluate powdered drugs with well-defined particles that can be counted, such as starch grains or single-layered cells or tissues, whose areas can be traced under the right magnification or objects of uniform thickness, whose

- The spores of lycopodium are very characteristic in shape and appearance and exceptionally uniform in size (about 25 μm).

- Quantitative microscopy is an analytical technique of great significance for powdered drugs, especially when chemical method of evaluation of crude drugs fail as accurate measure of quality.

- Lycopodium powder contains on an average 94,000 spores per mg.

- This method can be used to assess a powdered drug if it contains (i)well-defined particles that can be counted, such as pollen or starch grains, (ii)single-layered cells or tissues whose areas can be traced under the right magnification and their actual areas calculated, or (iii)uniform objects whose actual areas calculated.

Procedure for Lycopodium Spore Method

- Calculate the powdered material's loss on drying at 105°, Using a small, flexible spatula and a small amount of the suspending fluid, combine approximately 100 mg of the powdered medication and 50 mg of the lycopodium on a glass plate.

- Add enough suspending fluid (glycerine, tragacanth mucilage, water, or oil) to this combination to create a smooth, thin paste. Then, transfer the paste to a stoppered tube by washing it until 15 to 20 spores are visible in the field with a mm objective. For 50 mg of lycopodium, approximately 4 ml of the suspending agent is sufficient.

- Gently oscillate the stoppered container to ensure that the suspension is homogeneous. Apply the cover slip to both slides after placing one drop of the suspension on each, spread with a thin glass rod or needle, and lay aside for a few minutes on the table to allow the fluid mixture to settle properly. In each of the 25 observational fields, tally the ginger starch grains and the Lycopodium spores.

- Prepare another similar suspension and repeat the exercise.

- Form the mean of the 4 sets of the counts and percentage of moisture present, calculate the number of starch grains per mg, of the powder with reference to the powder dried at 105°.

- Pure Jamaica ginger contains 2 hundred 86 thousand starch grains per mg.

- Calculate the percentage purity of the ginger powder using the following formula:

N X W X 94,000 X A100 /S X M X P

Where,

N = number of starch grains in 25 fields,

W = weight in mg of lycopodium taken

S = number of spores in the same 25 fields

M = weight in mg of the sample, calculated on basis of sample dried at 105°,

P = 286,000

94,000 = number of lycopodium spores per mg.

Chemical Evaluation

- Chemical assays, quantitative chemical tests, qualitative chemical testing, and instrumental analysis are all included in the chemical evaluation.

- Chemical methods of evaluation include the isolation, purification, and identification of active components.

- Identification tests for numerous phytoconstituents such alkaloids, glycosides, tannins, etc. are included in qualitative chemical assays.

Examples:

Test for Alkaloids

A small amount (a few milligrammes) of each extract's residue was taken in 5 ml of 1.5% v/v hydrochloric acid and filtered separately. Alkaloid detection was then performed using these filtrates.

- Reddish brown precipitate is produced by Dragendorff's Reagent (potassium bismuth iodide solution).

- Mayer's Reagent, or potassium mercuric iodide solution, produces a precipitate that is cream in colour.

- Iodine-potassium iodide solution, or Wagner's Reagent, produces a reddish brown precipitate.

- Yellow precipitate results after using Hager's Reagent (picric acid solution).

Glycosides

A few chemical tests are:

Legal test

Add a few millilitres of pyridine, two drops of nitroprusside, and one drop of 20% sodium hydroxide solution to the medication. It turns a rich red colour.

Killer killiani test (test for deoxysugars)

A solution of 1% ferric sulphate solution and 5% glacial acetic acid is used to dissolve glycoside. One or two drops of strong sulfuric acid should be added. Deoxy sugar causes the development of a blue colour.

Baljet test

Add sodium picrate reagent to a piece of lamina or thick part of the leaf. Yellow to orange colour is visible if glycoside is present.

Borntrager's Test

Anthraquinones are detected using Borntrager's assay. The medication is cooked in diluted sulfuric acid, filtered, and then benzene, ether, or chloroform are added and vigorously agitated into the filtrate. After separating the organic layer, ammonia is gradually added to it. Due to the presence of anthraquinone glycosides, the ammonical layer is pink to red in hue.

Test for Sterols

Salkowski Test

A few mg of each extract's leftovers were placed in 2 ml of chloroform, to which 2 ml of concentrated sulfuric acid was poured from the test tube's side. Several minutes were spent shaking the test tube. Sterols are present when the chloroform layer turns red, which confirms their presence.

Liebermann-Burchard Reaction

Chloroform was used to dissolve a few milligrammes of residue. A few millilitres of acetic anhydride were added to this. Two drops of concentrated sulfuric acid were then introduced from the test tube's side. Sterols are present, as shown by the transitory greenish tint.

Test for Saponins

Foam Test

A test tube containing a few milligrammes of the test residue, some sodium bicarbonate, and water, was vigorously shaken. Saponins are present if stable, recognisable froth in the form of a honeycomb is produced.

Test for Tannins

Each extract's test residue was obtained separately, warmed in water, and filtered. Utilizing the filtrate as a test subject, the following reagent was used:

Ferric Chloride Test

It was created a 5% solution of ferric chloride in 90% alcohol. A few drops of this solution were added to the filtrate mentioned above. Tannins are present if a deep blue or dark green colour is achieved.

Lead Acetate Test

The test filtrate was mixed with a 10% w/v solution of basic lead acetate in distilled water. There are tannins present if precipitate is produced.

Potassium Dichromate Test

Tannins are present if, after adding a potassium dichromate solution to the test filtrate, a dark colour develops.

Test for Flavonoids

Shinoda Test

A little amount of test residue was dissolved in 5 ml of 95% v/v ethanol before being treated with 0.5 g of magnesium metal and a few drops of strong hydrochloric acid. If flavonoids are present, the pink, scarlet, or magenta colour develops within a minute or two.

Test for Proteins

Biuret Test

One millilitre of 4% copper sulphate was added to a few milligrammes of the residue that had been dissolved in water. Proteins cause a violet or pink hue to appear.

Xanthoprotein Test

2 ml of water and 0.5 ml of strong nitric acid were added to a little amount of residue. If there are proteins, a yellow colour results.

Test for Amino Acid

Ninhydrin Test

The ninhydrin reagent is a ninhydrin 0.1% w/v solution in n-butanol. The test extract was mixed with a small amount of this reagent. Amino acids cause the development of a violet or purple tint.

Test for Sugars

Molisch's Test

10 g of -naphthol were dissolved in 100 ml of 95% alcohol to create the Molisch's reagent. Two drops of Molisch's reagent were added to a test tube containing 0.5 ml of water and a few milligrammes of the test extract. 1 cc of concentrated sulfuric acid was introduced to this solution from the side of the inclined test tube, forming a layer beneath the aqueous solution without interacting with it. Sugars are present if a reddish-brown ring develops on the liquids' common surface.

Barfoed's Test

To make this reagent, 13.3 g of neutral copper acetate crystals were dissolved in 200 ml of a 1% acetic acid solution. When heated with a small amount of the reagent, the test residue was dissolved in water. Monosaccharides are present if a red cuprous oxide precipitate forms within two minutes.

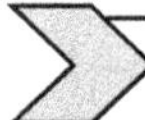 # Physical Evaluation

The physical parameter like solubility property, SG, OR, Viscosity, RI, MP, water content, degree of fibre elasticity, and other physical properties of the herb material are frequently assessed using physical methods in crude plant evaluation.

Solubility

Behaviors particular to drugs toward solvents are taken into account. This is helpful for looking at various oils, oleoresins, etc.

Examples

The solubility level of colophony in light petroleum, solubility property of balsam of Peru in chloral hydrate solution, the solubility of castor oil in half its volume of light petroleum, and the turbidity produced with two volumes of the solvent; Castor oil is soluble only in three volumes of 90% alcohol, while the adulterated form exhibits good solubility in alcohol.

Optical Rotation

Plane-polarized light can be rotated by anisotropic crystalline materials and samples with an excess of one enantiomer of a chiral chemical. Optically active compounds are those that exhibit the feature known as optical rotation. The dextrorotatory (d) or (+) enantiomer and the levorotatory (1) or (—) enantiomer are the two enantiomers that rotate light in opposite directions, or clockwise and counterclockwise, respectively, when viewed in the direction of light propagation.

Examples of drugs

Eucalyptus oil shows optical rotation around 0° to + 10°, honey shows at + 3° to —15° and Chenopodium oil at — 30° to — 80° etc.

Refractive Index (RI)

RI, is the difference between the speed of light in a vacuum and the speed of light passing via material is a feature of a material which alters the speed of light.

Their RI influence the angle of transmission, refracts the light beam when it passes through two different materials at an angle. Light generally has a refractive index that varies depending on its frequency, therefore colours of light move at different speeds. The refractive index can also be altered by high intensities.

Examples:

Castor oil 1.4758 to 1.527 and

Clove oil 1.527 to 1.535, etc.

Specific Gravity

It also goes by the name relative density. The ratio of solid or liquid mass to the mass of distilled water at 39°Fahrenheit or a gas to an equal volume of air or hydrogen under at specific temperature and pressure.

Examples:

Cottonseed oil 0.88-0.93,

Coconut oil 0.925 and castor oil 0.95.

Viscosity

The resistance of a fluid to flow is its viscosity. This resistance prevents both the movement of the fluid itself past immovable objects as well as the passage of any solid item through the fluid.

A liquid's viscosity, which serves as a gauge of its composition, is constant at a given temperature.

Internally, the fluid between neighbouring layers that move more slowly and more quickly is affected by viscosity. It serves as an evaluation parameter

Example: Liquid Paraffin NLT 64 centistokes at 37.8°C.

Melting Point

The temperature at which a solid transforms into a liquid is known as its melting point.

The melting points of plant components are exceedingly precise and constant. Due to chemical mixtures, the melting point range of crude pharmaceuticals has been fixed.

Examples: Melting point of beeswax is at 62-65°C, wool fat is at 34-44°C and agar melts at 85°C, etc.

Moisture Content

The amount of moisture in a medicine will determine whether it takes place chemically or by microbial development. Therefore, a drug's moisture content needs to be assessed and managed. By heating a medicine to a constant weight at 105°C in an oven, the moisture content can be calculated.

Examples: Digitalis and Ergot - NMT 5% w/w and 8% w/w.

Ultraviolet Light

When the tissue or powder is subjected to UV radiation, some medications glow, which is helpful in identifying those drugs. In powdered form, Indian and Chinese rhubarb can be quite challenging to differentiate from one another, however inspection under ultraviolet light reveals such pronounced variances in fluorescence that the types can be clearly identified from one another.

Ash Values

Ash analysis can be used to identify subpar goods, used-up medications, and an abundance of sand or other earthy materials. The detection of crude pharmaceuticals uses a variety of ash values, including total ash, acid-insoluble ash, watersoluble ash, and sulphated ash.

Total Ash

It is helpful in identifying illicit compounds that have been blended with other inorganic materials, such as nutmeg and ginger, to improve their look, such as sand, soil, calcium oxalate, or chalk powder.

Because higher temperatures would lose alkali chlorides that may be volatile, the maximum temperature employed for total ash should not be higher than 450°C.

Ash that is insoluble in diluted hydrochloric acid is known as acid-insoluble ash. It frequently has greater worth than the entire ash.

The amount of calcium oxalate in crude medications varies a great deal and is present in the majority of them.

As a result, for samples of genuine medicine, the total ash of a crude drug varies within large ranges.

Example: rhubarb, total ash range from 8 to 40%.

Acid insoluble ash

To find earthy stuff adhered to such a medication, the overall amount of ash is meaningless. So for rhubarb, acid insoluble ash would be preferred. When the ash is treated with HCl, the burned oxalate will produce calcium oxide or carbonate, which is soluble in the acid. The remaining ash, which is referred to as the acid-insoluble ash, is weighed. This allows us to identify the presence of too much earthy material, which is typical of roots and rhizomes.

Water soluble ash

Ash that dissolves in water is used to find materials that have been depleted by water. Sulphated ash is created by adding sulfuric acid to obtain sulphate salts, and the percentage of ash is estimated using the air-dried medication as a reference. This is done at a temperature greater than 600°C.

Examples:

The total ash value and water-soluble ash values of ginger are 6 and 1.7%, respectively.

Extractive Values

The extracts produced when crude pharmaceuticals are exhausted with various solvents are approximations of their chemical components. Depending on the sort of elements that need to be investigated different solvents are utilised. For crude drugs containing tannins, glycosides, mucilage and other water-soluble constituents an alcohol-soluble extractive is used. For drugs containing tannins, glycosides, resins, and other water-soluble constituents an ether-soluble extractive is used and for drugs containing volatile constituents and fats an ether-soluble extractive is used.

Foreign Organic Matter

Foreign organic matters are the organ or organ parts that aren't those that are listed in the definition and description of the medicine. They could be a bug, a mould, dirt, animal waste, etc. Every vegetable medication has its own limitations.

Examples:

Garlic should not contain MT 2% and Shatavari should not contain more than 1%.

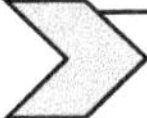 **Chromatography and Spectroscopical Techniques**

Paper Chromatography

- Paper chromatography is a type of planar chromatography in which the substances are separated using cellulose filter paper as a stationary phase. Partition chromatography, in which the compounds are spread or partitioned between liquid phases, is the underlying principle.

- Water is held in two phases: the stationary phase, which travels over the filter paper, and the mobile phase, which is held in the pores of the paper. When the mobile phase moves under the capillary action of paper pores, the compounds in the mixture separate as a result of variations in their affinities for water (in the stationary phase) and other solvents (in the mobile phase).

Thin Layer Chromatography

- Thin Layer Chromatography (TLC) is a solid-liquid method in which a solid (stationary phase) and a liquid are the two phases (moving phase). The two solids used in chromatography the most frequently are alumina and silica gel (SiO_2 x H_2O) (Al_2O_3 x H_2O).

- Thin Layer Chromatography (TLC) is an analytical method that is sensitive, quick, easy, and reasonably priced.

- In TLC, the sample to be examined is placed close to one end of a glass or plastic sheet that has been thinly covered with an adsorbent.

- In a closed jar with a thin coating of solvent, the sheet—which can be the size of a microscope slide—is laid on end.

- Differential partitioning between the components of the mixture dissolved in the solvent and the stationary adsorbent phase occurs as the solvent rises by capillary action up through the adsorbent.

- The stronger a given component of a mixture is adsorbed onto the stationary phase, the less time it will spend in the mobile phase and the slower it will migrate up the plate.

Applications

- The TLC method is effective for alkaloids, glycosides, isoprenoids, lipid components, sugars, and derivatives, and it has some advantages over paper chromatography.

- Finding contaminants in herbal medicines.

- It is quick, affordable, and easy to use.

- Several samples from several chemical races can be run at once with reliable standards.

Examples of phytoconstituents

Phyto-constituents	Plant product	Stationary phase	Mobile phase	Detection	R_f
18β Glycyrrhetinic acid	Liquorice formulation	Silica gel	Ethylacetate: Methanol: Ammonia (10:3:1)	Anisaldehyde Sulphuric acid reagent or 1% Vanillin Sulphuric acid reagent	**0.92**
Atropine	Atropa belladona	Silica gel	Toulene: Ethylacetate: Diethylamine (70:20:10)	Dragendroff's reagent	**0.70**
Menthol	Mentha piperata	Silica gel	Pure chloroform	1% vanillin – Sulphuric acid reagent. Heat at 110°C for 10min	**0.48 – 0.62**

Table *Contd...*

Phyto-constituents	Plant product	Stationary phase	Mobile phase	Detection	R_f
Carvone	Extract of Cuminum cyminum	Silica gel	Chloroform: acetone (100:2)	By dipping in anisaldehyde sulphuric acid Heat at 80°C for 10 minutes	**0.7517**
Aloin	Tincture of Aloe vera	Silica gel	Ethylacetate: Formic acid: Water (2:1:11)	Spraying with 10% sulphuric acid in alcohol heat at 100°C for 5 minutes	**0.47**
Caffeine	Coffee arabica	Silica gel	Ethylacetate: Methanol: acetic acid (80:10:10)	Expose to vapours of iodine	**0.41**
Reserpine	Rauwolfia serpentina	Silica gel	Chloroform: Acetone: diethylamine (50: 40:10)	Dragendroff's reagent	**0.72**

High Performance Thin Layer Chromatography

- HPTLC is a modern adaptation of TLC with better and advanced separation efficiency and detection limits.

- HPTLC is the most sophisticated type of TLC used today. It makes use of HPTLC plates with tiny particles and a restricted size distribution. Thus, uniform layers with a smooth surface are possible. HPTLC use smaller plates (10 10 or 10 20 cm), development distance is typically 6 cm, and analysis time is greatly reduced (7–20 min). HPTLC plates are utilised for industrial pharmaceutical densitometric quantitative analysis because they offer better resolution, greater detection sensitivity, and superior in situ quantification.

- The selection of mobile phase is based on adsorbent material used as stationary phase and physical and chemical properties of analyte.

Applications

- Capability to evaluate multicomponent crude samples;

- Simple separation procedures, especially when using colourful chemicals like berberine.

- A wide range of solvents are available for the HPTLC development because the mobile phases are completely evaporated before the detection step.

- Two-dimensional separations are simple to carry out. Multiple samples can be separated parallel to one another on the same plate, resulting in a high output, time savings, and a quick low-cost analysis.

- Specific and sensitive colour reagents can be used to detect separated spots like Dragendroff reagent/Kedde reagent.

- HPTLC can be combined and then used for several modes of evaluation, enabling the identification of substances with various light-absorption properties or various colours.

- The HPTLC approach may help to reduce the danger of exposure to harmful organic effluents and the difficulties associated with their disposal, hence minimising environmental contamination.

- It is also used to obtain fingerprint patterns of herbal formulations, quantification of active ingredients and also detection of adulteration crude drugs.

Examples of some herbal consistuents

Phyto-constituents	Plant product	Stationary phase	Mobile phase	Detection	Quantification
18β Glycyrrhetinic acid	Liquorice formulation	Silica gel	Ethylacetate: Methanol: Ammonia (10:3:1)	Anisaldehyde Sulphuric acid reagent or 1% Vanillin Sulphuric acid reagent	UV absorbance (densitometry) 260nm
Panaxadiol & Panaxatriol	Marked formulation of ginseng	Silica gel	Chloroform: ether (1:1)	Spraying 10% sulphuric acid in methanol Heat at 105°C for 10 minutes	UV absorbance (densitometry) 544nm and 52nm
Flavonol glycosides	Gingki biloba leaf extract	Silica gel	Chloroform: Benzene: Ethanol: Acetic acid: Water (11:4:2:1:2)	Spraying with 8% $AlCl_3$ in ethanol	UV absorbance (densitometry) 370nm
Carvone	Extract of Cuminum cyminum	Silica gel	Chloroform: acetone (100:2)	By dipping in anisaldehyde sulphuric acid Heat at 80°C for 10 minutes	UV absorbance (densitometry) 410nm
Aloin	Tincture of Aloe vera	Silica gel	Ethylacetate: Formic acid: Water (2:1:11)	Spraying with 10% sulphuric acid in alcohol heat at 100°C for 5 minutes	UV absorbance (densitometry) 350nm

Compilation of phytoconstituents profiles pertaining to varied range like opium alkaloids, anthraquinone derivatives like valtrate, rotenone, aristolchic acids, gibberellins, antibiotics and no of other compounds of natural origin.

Gas Liquid Chromatography

- Gas-liquid chromatography is a powerful tool in analysis.

- In gas-liquid chromatography, the mobile phase is a gas such as helium and the stationary phase is a high boiling point liquid adsorbed onto a solid.

- How fast a particular compound travels through the machine will depend on how much of its time is spent moving with the gas as opposed to being attached to the liquid in some way.

Applications

- Gas chromatography is a particularly essential tool for the investigation of volatile components in herbal medicines. The volatile oil analysis by GC has a lot of benefits. First, the volatile oil's GC analysis provides a reliable "fingerprint" that may be used to locate the plant.

- It is used to assay of starting materials and drug substances.

- Quantification of drug in formulations

- Assay of impurities or solvents in raw material and drug substances.

- Its important applications is to examine plant acids, alkaloids, resins glycosides, steroidal compounds and aminoacids etc.,

- Modification of sample structre may be accomplished by derivatization and mostly used derivatization is silylation.

- The most common derivatising agents used are trimethylchlorosilane, hexamethyldisilazone.

A few examples of phytoconstituents are:

Test Sample	Phytoconstituent	Gas Chromatography model	Column	Stationary phase	Carrier gas	Flow rate	Sample size	Column temperature
Eucalyptus oil	1,8 Cineole	NUCON 5765	Capillary 30m long fused silica column	FFAP (Free Fatty acid phase)	He	1.5ml/min	0.20µl	Isothermal 90°C/5 min
Clove oil	Eugenol	NUCON 5765	Capillary 30m long fused silica column	FFAP	He	1.5ml/min	0.20µl	Isothermal 90°C/2 min
Dill oil	Anethole	NUCON 5765	Capillary 30m long fused silica column	FFAP	He	1.5ml/min	0.20µl	Isothermal 100°C/2 min
Mint oil	1-Menthol	NUCON 5765	Capillary 30m long fused silica column	FFAP	He	1.5ml/min	0.20µl	Isothermal 100°C/2 min

- The moisture content determination in several plant drugs can be analyzed and identification of volatile terpenes is combined with TLC.

High Performance Liquid Chromatography

- The separation of the analyte in between a mobile phase and a stationary phase is the foundation of the HPLC separation principle.

- Depends on the chemical entity, the analyte consisting of molecules pass through the stationary phase more slowly.

- Different components of a sample are eluted at different periods because of the particular intermolecular interactions between the molecules of a sample and the packing material. In this way, the sample ingredients are successfully separated. After leaving the column, the analytes are recognised by a detecting unit.

- The signals are converted and recorded by a data management system and then shown in a chromatogram.

Applications

- Preparative and analytical HPLC are widely used in pharmaceutical industry for isolating and purification of herbal compounds.

- It helps to identify the various components present in the herbal product.

- This analysis tells you about the concentration of each component in the herbal product.

- It assesses the purity of the herbal product.

- HPLC analysis in combination with Evaporative Light Scattering Detection method help in the analysis of non- chromophoric compounds.

- The versatility of this method for analysis of chemical compounds in herbal drugs makes it the most preferred method to assess the quality of the herbal drugs.

- This method must be inculcated in the protocol of all herbal testing laboratories to increase the efficacy of herbal treatments.

- A few examples of phytoconstituents are:

Herbal drug extract	Active compounds	Column	Mobile phase	Flow rate	Gradient	Detector	Stop time	Inj vol.
Atropa Belladona	Atropine	4.6 × 75 mm Zorbax Eclipse XDB-C18, 3.5 µm	A = 0.05 M KH2P04 in water (pH = 3), B = acetonitrile	1.0 ml/min	At 0 min 10% B At 20 min 60% B At 23 min 60% B At 25 min 10% B	UV [diode array detector 210 nm/16 (ref. 360 nm/100), standard cell]	25 min	5 µl
Cortex Cinchonae	Quinidine Quinine	4 × 125 mm Purospher RP- 18,5 µm	A = 0.05 M KH2P04 in water (pH = 3), B = acetonitrile	0.8 ml/min	At 0 min 4% B At 25 min 10% B At 45 min 30% B At 46 min 60% B At 49 min 60% B At 50 min 4% B	UV [diode array detector 210 nm/16 (ref. 360 nm/100), standard cell]	50 min	5 µl
Ephedra Sinica	Ephedrine Norephedrine	4.6 × 75 mm Zorbax SB- C18, 3.5 µm	A = 0.025 M KH2P04 in water (pH = 3), B = acetonitrile	1.0 ml/min	At 0 min 2% B At 10 min 10% B At 15 min 80% B At 18 min 80% B At 20 min 2% B	UV [diode array detector 210 nm/16 (ref. 360 nm/100), standard cell]	20 min	5 µl
Ginko Biloba	Quercetin Kaempferol	4 × 125 mm Hypersil ODS, 5 µm	A = 0.5% H 3P04 in water, B = methanol	2.0 ml/min	At 0 min 38% B At 12 min 48% B At 17 min 100% B At 20 min 38% B	Diode array detector 370 nm/16 (ref. off), standard cell	20 min	10 µl
Rheum Palmatum	Rhein Emodin	4 × 125 mm Hypersil ODS, 5 µm	A = 0.05 M NH4 0Ac in water (pH = 2.5), B = acetonitrile	1.0 ml/min	At 0 min 30% B At 10 min 80% B At 14 min 80% B At 15 min 30% B	Diode array detector 440 nm/16 (ref. off), standard cell	15 min	1 µl

Column Chromatography

Adsorption of a solution's solutes through a stationary phase, which separates the mixture into its component parts, is the primary principle of column chromatography. The affinity for the mobile phase and stationary phase is the foundation for this. More and less affine molecules elute at different times, with more affine molecules eluting later and less affine molecules eluting first.

Applications

Similar to HPLC but column is packed with silica gel slurry by wet packing or dry packing.

Spectrophotometric Methods

UV and Visible Spectroscopy

- Ultraviolet-visible spectroscopy is considered an important tool in analytical chemistry.

- Spectroscopy has to do with how light and matter interact. The amount of energy in the atoms or molecules increases as light is absorbed by matter. An identifiable spectrum results from a chemical substance absorbing visible light or ultraviolet radiation.

- The region from 190 to 380nm is known as UV region and from 380 – 900nm is known as Visible region.

Applications

1. It is among the best techniques for identifying contaminants. Impurities can be identified by looking for additional peaks that are caused by the sample's impurities, comparing the observed peaks to those of a standard raw material, and measuring the absorbance at a particular wavelength.

2. It is useful in the structure elucidation of phytconstituents such as the presence of heteroatoms.

3. UV absorption spectroscopy can be used for the quantitative determination of compounds that absorb UV radiation.

4. It helps to determine the quality of chemicals. By contrasting the absorption spectrum with the spectra of recognised substances, identification is accomplished.

5. This method is used to determine whether a functional group is present in the chemical or not. The lack of a band at a specific wavelength is seen as proof that a certain group does not exist.

6. UV spectroscopy can also be used to study reaction kinetics.

7. Many medications are either available as raw materials or as finished products. By preparing a suitable drug solution in a solvent and detecting the absorbance at a particular wavelength, they can be tested.

8. Compounds' molecular weights can be determined spectrophotometrically by making the appropriate derivatives of these compounds.

9. An HPLC detector that uses a UV spectrophotometer is possible.

Some of the Examples are:

S. No.	Natural Products	Maximum wavelength
1.	Lobeline	249
2.	Reserpine	268
3.	Morphine	286
4.	Vanillin	301
5.	Morphine	442
6.	Cardioactive glycosides	590
7.	Anthraquinone	505

UV radiation tests for natural products

S. No.	Natural Products	1N HCl
1.	Almond	Dull blue green
2.	Black pepper	Blue
3.	Cardamom	Brownish green
4.	Fennel	Bluish green
5.	Linseed	Greenish blue
6.	Physostigma	Blue
7.	Thyme	Brownish green

Infra Red Spectroscopy

- The idea that molecules prefer to absorb particular light frequencies that are distinctive of the corresponding structure of the molecules underlies the IR spectroscopy theory. The energies depend on the atomic mass, the related vibronic coupling, and the geometry of the molecular surfaces.

- For instance, the molecule may be able to absorb the energy present in the incident light, which will cause it to rotate more quickly or vibrate more loudly.

- The IR region is divided into 3 regions viz., 12500-4000 cm^{-1} (Near IR) 4000-400 cm^{-1} and 400-20 cm^{-1}.

- Mid IR Region is widely used for the analysis of drugs and pharmaceuticals.

Applications

- It is used in identification of substances by comparing identical IR spectra of sample and standard.
- Small difference in structure and constitution of molecule result in significant changes in the peaks in this region. Hence this region helps to identify an unknown compound.
- Determination of Molecular Structure
- Detection of Impurities which is determined by comparing sample spectrum with the spectrum of pure reference compound.
- Isomers can be identified.
- Identification of Functional Groups Due to the presence of functional group region.
- To Determine impurities in raw materials (to ensure quality products).
- For Quality Control checks; to determine the % of required product.

Flourescence Analysis

- Fluorescence spectrometry is a quick, easy, and affordable way to gauge an analyte's concentration in a solution based on its fluorescence characteristics.
- When the type of compound to be examined (the "analyte") is known, it can be used for relatively straightforward analyses to perform a quantitative analysis to ascertain the concentration of the analytes.
- Fluorescence is mostly used to measure substances in solution.

Nuclear Magnetic Resonance Spectroscopy

Numerous nuclei have spin, and all nuclei are electrically charged, according to the NMR underlying principle.

An energy transition from the base energy to a higher energy level is achievable in the presence of an external magnetic field.

When the spin returns to its base level, an emission at the same frequency occurs. The energy transfer occurs at a wavelength that corresponds to radio frequencies.

To produce an NMR spectrum for the target nucleus, the signal that corresponds to this transfer is measured in various ways and using various procedures.

Applications

- Molecular structure, content, and purity of a sample are all determined using this analytical chemistry approach, which is also employed in research to control the quality of herbal medications.

- For instance, mixtures containing known substances can be quantitatively analysed using NMR.

- It makes use of straightforward one-dimensional approaches to explore chemical structure. The structure of more complex molecules is determined via two-dimensional methods.

- These methods are taking the place of x-ray crystallography in the analysis of protein structure.

Mass Spectroscopy

- Mass spectrometry is a potent analytical method used to determine the structure and chemical characteristics of various molecules, identify unknown chemicals within a sample, and quantify recognised materials.

- The material is transformed into gaseous ions throughout the entire process, either with or without fragmentation, and these ions are then classified according to their relative abundances and mass to charge ratios (m/z).

- This method essentially investigates how molecules are affected by ionising energy. The consumption of sample molecules during the creation of ionic and neutral species depends on chemical events occurring in the gas phase.

Applications

- MS has become a powerful tool in proteomics research. It helps in Protein identification, Protein Quantification.

- Post-translational modifications:

- Post Translational Modifications are chemical alterations to protein structure.

- Mass Spectrometry in Metabolomics. MS is commonly used analytical tools for small-molecule analysis in metabolomics.

- Mass spectrometry imaging (MSI) is a technology to visualize the spatial distribution of molecules.

A few Examples are

- Zeatin, a first naturally occur cytokinin growth hormone shows a prominent molecular ion at 219 confirming the molecular formula $C_{10}H_{13}ON_5$.

- Atropine shows a prominent peak at 124 confirming the molecuarl formula as $C_{17}H_{23}NO_3$.

- Quinine shows a prominent peak at 136 confirming the molecular formula as $C_{20}H_{24}N_2O_2$.

- Reserpine shows peak at 195,251,397,607 & 608 confirming the molecular formulas $C_{33}H_{40}N_2O_9$.

- Diosgenin shows a prominent peak at 415 confirming the molecular formula $C_{27}H_{42}O_3$.

- Ephedrine shows a peak at 148,166,167 confirming the molecular formula as $C_{10}H_{15}NO$.

Biological Evaluation

Evaluation of antidiabetic activity

(a) Streptozocin induced diabetic model

- Healthy albino Wistar rats of both sexes weighing about 150-250 g were taken.

- There were four groups of six animals each (n = 6) made up of the animals. Group I acted as the control and received distilled water; Group II was given the standard medication (10 mg/kg body weight); and Groups III and IV underwent tests using the minimum and maximum doses. The rats underwent an overnight fast before being given oral glucose (2 g/kg body weight) 30 min following treatment to determine their tolerance to the substance. After administering glucose, blood glucose levels were measured at 0, 30, 60, and 120 minutes.

- STZ was used to cause diabetes at a dose of 40 mg/kg body weight. To prepare the medication, it was newly dissolved in 0.1 M citrate buffer (pH 4.5). Rats that had been fasting for the previous night were then given the solution intraperitoneally. The rats were tested for diabetes after 72 hours, and those with fasting blood glucose (FBG) levels under 200 mg/dL were diagnosed.

- After induction the treatment was carried out for 6 weeks. After 6 weeks the blood samples were collected from caudal vein tested for biochemical parameters.

(b) In order to determine each group's level of diabetes, biochemical parameters were examined. Blood glucose levels were monitored weekly at intervals of 0 days, 7 days, and 14 days after the daily administration of extract orally.

(c) After each animal was sacrificed under anaesthesia, the entire pancreas was taken for histopathological investigations. The pancreas was fixed in neutral formalin fixative solution at 10% for a portion of it. Tissues were fixed, embedded in paraffin, thick slices were cut at 4-5 m, and stained for histological analysis using hematoxylin and eosin. Light microscopy examination of the slices was done.

(d) Alloxan induced diabetic model:

- Healthy albino Wistar rats of both sexes weighing about 150-250 g were taken.

- The animals were divided into four groups of six animals ($n = 6$) each. Group I served as control and received distilled water; Group II received Standard drug (10 mg/kg body weight); Group III & IV test plant of minmal and maximal dose. The rats were on overnight fast and glucose tolerance was tested by oral administration of glucose (2 g/kg body weight) to normoglycemic rats 30 min after treatment. Blood glucose levels were estimated at 0 min, 30 min, 60 min, and 120 min after glucose administration.

- The Diabetes was induced using alloxan at a dose of 100 mg/kg body weight. The drug was freshly prepared by dissolving in normal saline. The solution was then administered intraperitoneally to rats that had been on overnight fast prior to administration. After 72 h the animals were screened for diabetes, and the rats that showed fasting blood glucose (FBG) $\geq$200 mg/dL.

- After induction the treatment was carried out for 6 weeks.After 6 weeks the blood samples were collected from caudal vein tested for biochemical parameters.

- Biochemical parameters were studied i.e., Blood glucose was measured using one touch glucometer at weekly intervals, that is, 0 days, 7 days, and 14 days after the daily administration of extract orally to ascertain the diabetic status of each group.

- Histopathological studies were carried out by taking up the whole pancreas from each animal was removed after sacrificing under anesthesia. A portion of the pancreas was fixed in 10% neutral formalin fixative solution. After fixation, tissues were embedded in paraffin; thick sections were cut at 4-5 μm and stained with hematoxylin and eosin for histological examinations. The sections were examined under light microscope.

Hepatoprotective Activity

Carbon tetrachloride Induced liver Fibrosis in rats

- Albino rats were selected for the study and treated with ccl4 dissolved in oil (1:1).

- Animals were grouped into 4 i.e., control group, group treated with CCL4, and test treated group and standard group.

- Animal weight is tested weekly.

- After 8 weeks of treatment the animals were anaesthetised and the serum is evaluated for Bilirubin and bile acids.

- After 8 weeks the animals were crucified. The liver sections were made and observed under microscope for the development of fibrosis.

- If it is 0:Normal, I: Tiny, II: Large Septa, III: Nodular Transformation & IV: Excessive formation.

Paracetomol model

- Mice is taken for this model. All the mices were given paracetomol 500mg/kg for the induction of heptotoxicity.

- After 48hr the treatment was given for 5 days with test drug.

- After 5 days bilirubin, creatinine levels were checked and histopathaological studies were carried out by preparing liver sections and observed under microscope for the development of fibrosis.

- If it is 0:Normal, I: Tiny, II: Large Septa, III: Nodular Transformation & IV: Excessive formation.

Antiulcer Activity

Pylorus ligation in rats

Wistar rats weighing 150–225 g were employed in the investigation. Animals were kept in controlled environments with a temperature of 22 °C, relative humidity of 44% to 56%, and a 12-hour light/12-hour dark cycle.

The animals were divided into twelve groups, consisting of six each. Group I represented the normal control group, Group II represented the ulcerated control group, Group III represented the standard group,. Groups IV& V recieves test compound of two different doses, for 7 days.

Animals in all groups received 200 mg/kg of aspirin orally every day from days 5 to 7, two hours following the administration of each medication treatment.

Animals in each group were fasted for 18 hours following the allocated treatment before being put under anaesthesia. The rats were slaughtered, their stomachs were taken out, and they were checked for ulcers four hours after the pylorus was tied.

Ulcer score: Using magnifying glasses, the number of ulcers was counted. The diameter of each ulcer was then measured using a vernier calliper. The ulcer index was calculated using

$$\% \text{ Protection} = \frac{(\text{UI control} - \text{UI treated}) \times 100}{\text{UI control}}$$

Where UI stands for ulcer index.

Score board:

    0: No ulcers.

    1: Superficial Ulcers.

    2: Deep Ulcers.

    3: Perforations.

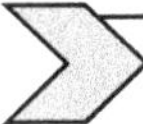

CHAPTER 4

Secondary Metabolites

Alkaloids

These are organic products from natural or synthetic origin which is basic in nature contains 1 or more nitrogen normally heterocyclic nature possess specific physiological action on human or animal body in lower dose.

Occurrence and Distribution

A total of 6000 structurally distinct alkaloids have been identified. The majority of them are found in flora, 1% in mammals, and less than 0.5 percent in fungi and bacteria. Botanists believe that there are about 20,000 plant genera. Only 9% of all genera have species that contain alkaloids. These alkaloid-containing plants are not evenly distributed among genera; rather, they are most prevalent in genera belonging to the Angiospermae's Dicotyledones and Monocotyledones (flowering plants). Alkaloids are uncommon in the Gymnospermae and Pteridophytae families.

According to some estimates, at least one alkaloid-containing species can be found in 40% of all plant families. On the other hand, some plant families (such as the Papaveraceae) include alkaloids in all of their species. As a result, the distribution of alkaloids in flora is extremely diverse.

Alkaloids can be found in a variety of plant parts, including the roots, stem, bark, leaves, fruits, and seeds. Alkaloids are separated from all parts of some plants (e.g., *Papaver somniferum, A. belladonna*), whereas they are found in only one portion of others (e.g., the alkaloid of *Aphelandra squarrosa* is only found in the roots).

The amount of structurally distinct alkaloids differs between plants. *Catharanthus roseus*, for example, contains over 100 alkaloids. The composition of an alkaloid combination is frequently variable in different regions of the plant. The age of the plant (e.g., *Adhatoda vasica*), the season (e.g., *P. somniferum*), the gathering time of the day (e.g., Conium maculatum), and the habitat are all factors that influence the level and diversity of alkaloid content (e.g., *Maytenus buxifolia*). The total amount of alkaloids in plants varies between ten percent of quinine (*Cinchona sp.*) and ten percent of the drug's dried weight.

Isolation of Alkaloids

Alkaloids can be extracted by direct crystallization from solvent, steam distillation, chromatographic techniques and Gradient pH technique.

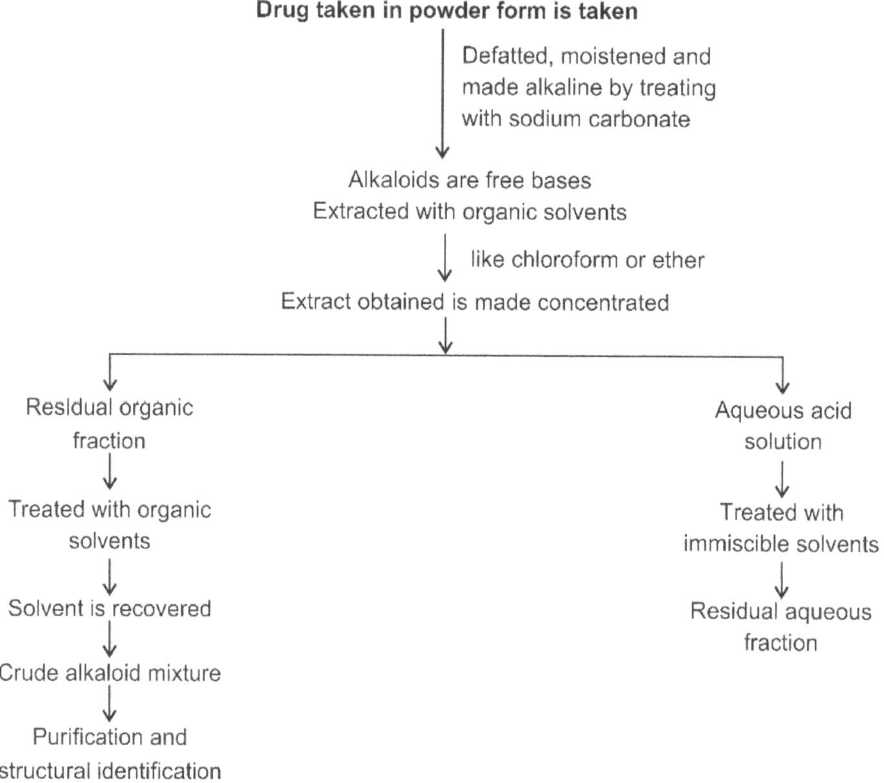

Drug taken in powder form is taken

General Identification Tests

- **Mayers Reagent:** Alkaloids are treated with Potassium Mercuric Iodide gives cream colored precipitate.

- **Dragendroff reagent:** Alkaloids are treated with Potassium Bismuth Iodide gives reddish brown colored precipitate.

- **Wagners Reagent:** Alkaloids are treated with Iodine Potassium Iodide gives cream colored precipitate.

- **Hagers Reagent:** Alkaloids are treated with Picric acid gives yellow colored precipitate.

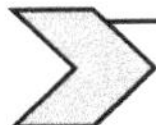 ## Therapeutic activity and Pharmaceutical Applications

A few examples are noted here:

S. No.	Crude Drug	Chemical Constituents	Therapeutic activity and Pharmaceutical Applications
Ergot alkaloids			
1.	Ergot	Ergometrine, Ergotamine	Treatment of migraine, oxytocic activity
2.	Nux vomica	Strychnine, brucine	CNS Stimulant
3.	Vinca	Vincristine, vinblastine	Antineoplastic
Isoquinoline alkaloids			
4.	Opium	Narcotine, papaverine	Analgesic
Tropane alkaloids			
5.	Belladonna	Hyoscyamine, atropine	Anticholinergic, antispasmodic
6.	Datura	Scopolamine, Hyoscyamine, atropine	Anticholinergic, duodenal ulcers
Quinoline alkaloids			
7.	Cichona	Quinine, quinidine, cinchonine and cinchonidine	Antimalarial
Purine alkaloids			
8.	Coffee	caffeine	Stimulant
Imidazole alkaloids			
9.	Pilocarpus	Pilocarpine, pilosine	Cholinergic, treatment of glaucoma
Steroidal alkaloids:			
10.	Ashwagandha	Withanine, withaferine	Antirheumatic, sedative.

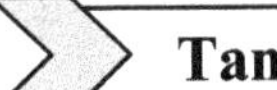 ## Tannins

- These are the secondary metabolites which is in the form of a solution in cell sap or distinct vacuoles.
- They are known as astringents from longtime.
- Tannins are used in leather industry to prevent Putrefaction. Putrefaction is the final stage of death or decomposition.
- They are chemically complex organic substances contains polyphenols.
- They have high molecular weight.
- They are devoid of Nitrogen
- They are non-crystalline substances.

Occurrence and Distribution

Tannins can be found in plants from all over the world. Gymnosperms and angiosperms are both known to have them. The distribution of tannin in 180 dicotyledon families and 44 monocotyledon groups. Tannin-free species can be found in the majority of dicot groups. Aceraceae, Actinidiaceae, Anacardiaceae, Bixaceae, Myricaceae etc., for dicots, and Najadaceae and Typhaceae for monocots are the most well-known families in which all species examined contain tannin. Seventy-three percent of the plants evaluated in the oak family, Fagaceae, contain tannin. Condensed tannins are the most abundant polyphenols, occurring in practically all plant groups and accounting for up to 50% of the dry weight of leaves.

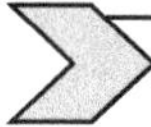

Isolation

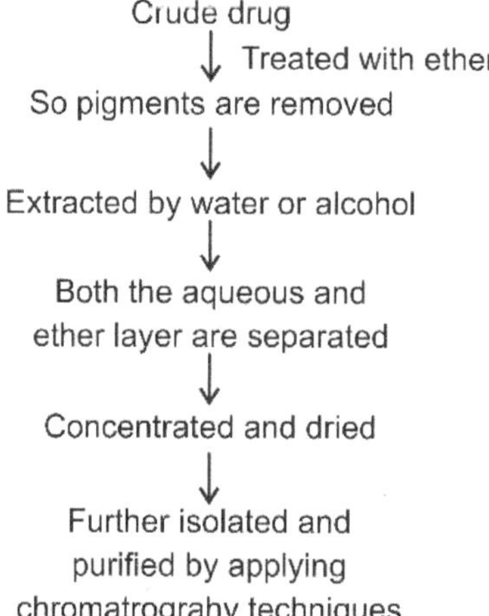

General Identification Tests

- It precipitates alkaloids & gelatine.
- Tannins are precipitated by salts of Cu, Sn & Pb.
- Tannins are precipitated by chromic acid solution.
- Tannins are precipitated by $FeCl_3$ is bluish black or brownish green color.

- **Gold beaters skin test:**

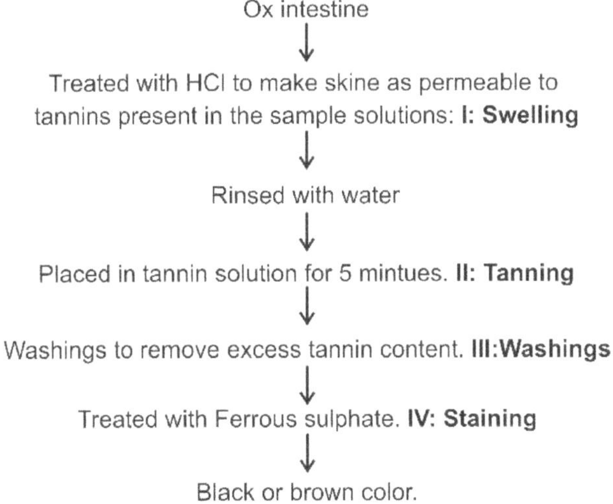

Therapeutic activity and Pharmaceutical Applications

A few examples are noted here

S. No.	Crude Drug	Chemical Constituents	Therapeutic activity and Pharmaceutical Applications
Hydrolysable Tannins:			
1.	Amla	Vitamin C, Phyllemblin and tannins	Diuretic, laxative and it is in composition of Triphala and chyavanprash
2.	Arjuna	Ellagic acid, beta-sitosterol	Cardiotonic, hypotensive.
3.	Myrobalan	Chebulic acid, Chebulagic acid, Gallic acid	Astringent, stomachic, purgative, ingredient in Triphala Churna.
Non-hydrolysable Tannins:			
4.	Ashoka	Catechin, Ketosterol	Uterine tonic and oxytocic
5.	Black Catechu	Acacatechin, quercetin	Astringent, skin eruptions.
6.	Pale Catechu	Catechin, Catechutannic acid	Astringent in the treatment of diarrhoea.

Terpenoids

Terpenoids

- Terpene is the term known as mixture of isomeric hydrocarbons.
- Terpene represents only hydrocarbons $(C_5H_8)_n$.
- Terpenoids represent hydrobcarbons as well as the oxygenated derivatives i.e., $(C_5H)_n$.

- All terpernes are terpenoids but not viceversa.
- On thermal decomposition it yields isoprene units.

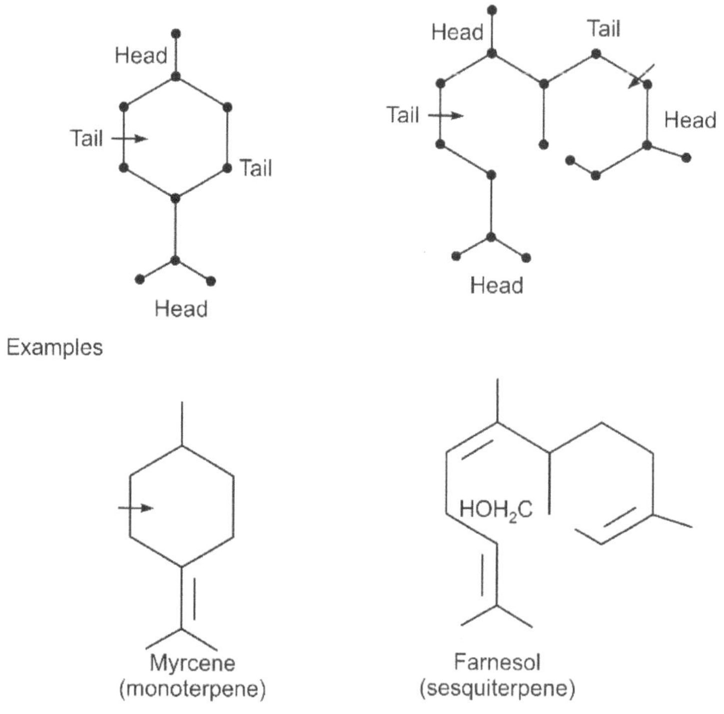

- All terpenoids is their derivation from one monomeric structural unit "Isoprene".
- In terpenoids isoprene units are attached to another moiety in Head & Tail arrangement Known as Special Isoprene Rule.

Special Isoprene Rule

Occurrence and Distribution

Plant terpenoids are employed in traditional herbal medicines for their fragrant properties. The aroma of eucalyptus, the flavours of cinnamon, cloves, and ginger, the golden colour of sunflowers, and the red colour of tomatoes are all terpenoids. Citral, menthol, camphor, salvinorin A in the herb Salvia divinorum, cannabinoids in cannabis, and ginkgolide and bilobalide in Ginkgo biloba are all examples of well-known terpenoids. The provitamin beta carotene is a carotenoid, which is a terpene derivative.

Terpenoids, also known as isoprenoids, natural compounds that play critical functions in all organisms' metabolism. Chemical variety of terpenoid metabolites is especially high in plants, where many are secondary metabolites. Many ecological interactions between plants and animals are mediated by non-essential, specialised plant terpenoids, which operate as to attract pollinators or repel herbivores. The recruitment of genes from primary metabolism hastened the evolution of terpenoid secondary metabolism in plants, which was aided by the proliferation of cytochrome P450 and terpenes synthase gene families in plant genomes. Terpenoid chemical variety reflects a natural history highlighted by herbivory stress and other animal-imposed selective pressures, resulting in a diverse range of synthesised terpenoids in the plant kingdom that are pre-selected for specific functions.

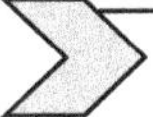 **Isolation of Terpenoids**

Drug
↓
Subjected for distillation to extract
mono and sesquiterpenoids
↓
Physical and chemical methods were applied
↓
Further, distillation under reduced pressure
and column chromatographic techniques were
employed to isolate terpenoids by properly
selecting the relevant adsorbent.

General Identification tests:

1. **Liebermann-Burchard test:** When chloroform solution of test sample is treated with acetic anhydride and concentrated sulphuric acid, green colour is formed due to the presence of terpenoids.

2. **Salkowski test:** When chloroform solution of test sample is treated with concentrated sulphuric acid, red colour is formed.

3. **Sulphur Powder Test:** The drug is treated with sulfur, sulfur is sinked in the mixture.

4. Colored precipitation is resulted when treated with *Trichloroacetic acid Test.*

5. Yellow precipitation is observed when treated with *Tetranitro Methane Test.*

6. **Zimmermann Test:** When the alcoholic solution of drug is treated with dinitrobenzene solution, made alkali results in violet color.

Therapeutic activity and Pharmaceutical Applications

A few examples are noted here:

S. No.	Crude Drug	Chemical Constituents	Therapeutic activity and Pharmaceutical Applications
Monoterpenoids			
1.	Cinnamon	Eugenol, benzaldehyde, cuminaldehyde	Carminative, stomachic, stimulant, aromatic,antiseptic and astringent.
2.	Corinader	Coriandrol, coriandryl acetate	Carminative
3.	Caraway	Carvone, carvacrol	Aromatic, carminative, stimulant
Sesquiterpenoids			
4.	Sandalwood oil	Santalol, santene, santalene	Treatment of dysuria, used in perfume.
5.	Clove	Eugenl, eugenin	Analgesic, Carminative, stimulant, aromatic and antiseptic.
Diterpenoids			
6.	Taxus	Taxol, deacetyl baccatin	anticancer
Triterpenoids			
7.	Ambergris	Ambrene	Perfumes
Tetraterpenoids and polyterpenoids			
8.	Crocus	Crocin, crocetin and picrocrocin	Antispasmodic, emmenagogue and stimulant.

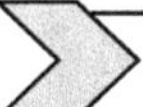

Volatile Oils

- Volatile principles of plants or animals are called volatile oils.
- When exposed to air they get evaporated at ordinary temperature hence called ethereal oils.
- They represent essence or active constituent of plant hence they are known as essential oils.
- They are derived from terpenoids.
- They are made up of isoprene units.
- They are soluble in alcohol, ether and insoluble in water.
- They possess characteristic odor.

- They have high Refractive Index and optically active.
- They are secreted in special structures called ducts, trichomes or schizogenous glands.
- They are extracted by Steam Distillation, Effluerage & Ecuelle.
- They are used as flavouring and perfuming agents.
- They are stored in well closed container, away from light and in cool place.

Occurrence and Distribution

It is widely distributed and occurred in families like Labiatae, Rutaceae etc., The volatile oil is present through out the plant or any part.

Extraction

1. Method of Expression

The plant material is crushed, and the juice is filtered to remove big particles. When almost half of the essential oil is extracted, the screening juice is centrifuged in a high-speed centrifugal machine. The remaining half of the oil is usually not extracted, and the residue is used for distillation to isolate inferior quality oil. This process is used to extract citrus, lemon, and grass oils.

2. Steam distillation Method

This is the most common approach; the plant material is macerated and then steam distilled, resulting in a distillate from which the essential oils can be extracted using pure organic volatile solvents such as light petroleum. However, because some essential oils are destroyed during distillation and others (esters) are hydrolyzed to none or less fragrant molecules, the process should be used with caution.

3. Extraction with a Volatile Solvent

Because some essential oils are heat sensitive and degrade during distillation, the plant material is immediately treated with light petrol at 50°C, and the solvent is extracted by distillation under reduced pressure.

4. Effleurage

Warm the fat on glass plates to around 50°C, then cover it with the petals (part of the flower) and leave it that way over several months until the fat is saturated with essential oils, at which point the old petals can be replaced with new ones. When the essential oils found in the fat are dissolved in ethyl alcohol, the petal is removed and the fat is digested with ethyl alcohol. If any fat is also dissolve during digestion, it is removed by chilling to about 20°C. To eliminate the solvent, the extract containing ethyl alcohol & essential oils is distillation under decreased pressure.

General Tests for Volatile oils

- To the section, add alcoholic solution of Sudan III gives red color.
- To the section, add tincture alkane gives red color.
- Evaporation on filter paper.

Therapeutic activity and Pharmaceutical Applications

A few examples are noted here:

Alcohol volatile oils – Sandalwood, Peppermint, Coriander etc.,

Aldehyde volatile oils – Cinnamon, Lemon peel, Citronella etc.,

Ester Volatile ois – Lavender, Mustard

Hydrocarbon volatile oils – Turpentine, Black pepper

Oxide volatile oils – Eucalyptus

Phenol volatile oils – Clove, Thyme etc.,

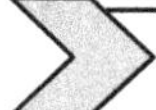

Resins

- Resins are amorphous substance.
- These are mixture of essential oil and oxygenated products with terpenes & carboxylic acid.
- They are translucent solids, semi-solids, or liquid substances.
- They are heavier than water which becomes soft when heated.
- They are electrically non-conductive.
- These are end products of metabolism which stores in schizogenous ducts or glands.
- They are chemically organic acids or alcohols or esters and neutral resins.
- They are insoluble in water partially in light petroleum.

Type of Constituent

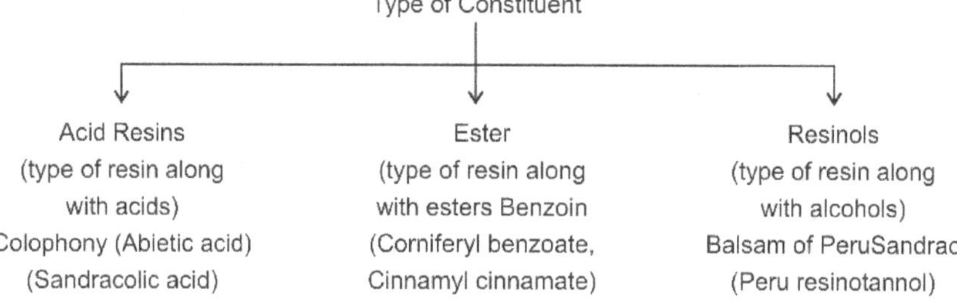

	Type of Constituent	
Acid Resins (type of resin along with acids) Colophony (Abietic acid) (Sandracolic acid)	Ester (type of resin along with esters Benzoin (Corniferyl benzoate, Cinnamyl cinnamate)	Resinols (type of resin along with alcohols) Balsam of PeruSandrac (Peru resinotannol)

Types of resins:

Resins + oils $\longrightarrow$ Oleoresins. Ex: Canada balsan

Oleo+ gum+ resins $\longrightarrow$ Oleogumresins. Ex: Myrrh

Resins + Sugars $\longrightarrow$ Glycoresins. Ex: Jalap

Resin + Balsamic & Cinnamic acid $\longrightarrow$ Balsams

Resenes: These are complex natural substances without any specific chemical properties and they are inert chemically. Ex:Asafoetida.

General Identification Test

1. HCl Test: Resins turns pink color when treated with HCl test.

2. $FeCl_3$ Test: Resins turns greenish blue color when treated with $FeCl_3$.

3. Umbelliferone test: Resins when treated with HCl, concentrated Ammonium hydroxide, $HNO_3.H_2SO_4$ and washed with water give blue flourescence, green, red and violet color.

4. Copper acetate test: Resins treated with petroleum give emerald green color.

Isolation of Resins

Because of the availability of diverse combinations, isolating resin from crude medicine might be a tough undertaking. However, the most widely used method is to extract the drug with alcohol, the precipitated the resin is mixed with a significant amount of water.

Therapeutic activity and Pharmaceutical Applications

A few examples are noted here:

S. No.	Crude Drug	Chemical Constituents	Therapeutic activity and Pharmaceutical Applications
1.	Asafoetida	Asaresinotannol	Carminative, nervine stimulant, intestinal flatulence.
2.	Benzoin	Benzoic acid and cinnamic acid and their esters, sumaresinolic & Siraresinolic acid	Expectorant, carminative, antiseptic.
3.	Ginger	Zingiberene, curcumene, gingerol, shogoals, gingediols	Carminative, flavouring agent, motion sickness.
4.	Myrrh	Commiphoric acids	Antiseptic, stimulant.
5.	Toly balsam	Cinammic acid, benzoic acid, benzoyl benzoate, toluresinotannol	Expectorant, flavouring agent.

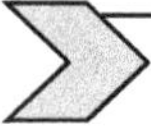 # Glycosides

Glycosides are the organic compounds from plant or animal sources which on enzymatic or acid hydrolysis gives one or more sugar moieties and non-sugar moiety exerts therapeutic activity.

Occurrence and Distribution

Glycosides are abundant in nature. It is widely distributed in some Scrophulareaceae - *Digitalis purpurea* and *Digitalis lanata, Picrorhiza kurroa,* Apocyanaceae - *Nerium oliander* and *Thevetia peruviana,* Liliacea - *Urgenea indica* and *U. maritima, Aloe vera, Leguminocae – Cassia acutefolia* and *C. angustefolia, Gly-cyrrhiza glabra, Psoralea corylifolia,* Dioscoreaceae *Dioscorea floribunda,* Rosaceae - *Prunus amygdalus, Carategus oxycantha etc., It is also well distributed among families Cruciferae, Gentianaceae, Acanthaceae, Simarubaceae, Umbelliferae, Rutaceae, Polygonaceae and Myrtaceae.*

Isolation of Glycosides

Stass-Otto Process

A method of extraction of alkaloids from plants and animal bodies: the substance is digested in alcohol and tartaric acid, the fatty and resinous matters are precipitated with water, the fluid is made alkaline, and the alkaloids are extracted with ether or chloroform.

Stass-Otto Process:

Powdered drug is taken

↓

Extract by Soxhlet apparatus by using solvent as alcohol

↓

The obtained extract is treated with lead acetate to precipitate tannins

↓

Excess lead acetate is precipitated as lead sulphide by hydrogen
sulphide gas through the solution

↓

The extract lead acetate is filtered, concentrated to get crude glycosides

↓

Further fractional crystallization and purification by chromatographic techniques.

General Identification Tests

Cardiac glycosides:

Keller-Killiani Test

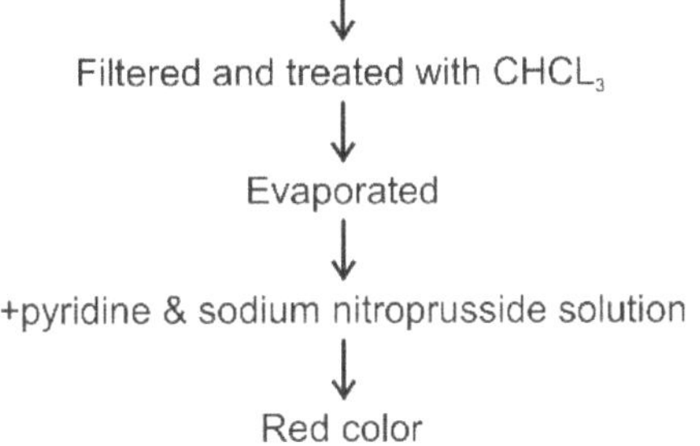

Legal test

Baljet Test

Anthraquinone glycosides

Borntragers test

The drug is powdered and extracted with ether. The filtered ethereal extract is made alkaline with caustic soda. Aqueous layer shows after shaking pink, red or violet color.

Modified Borntragers test

For anthranols borntragers test will give negative report hence modified borntragers test is perfomed. Take 0.1 gm of medication and combine it with 5 mL of ferric chloride 5 percent solution and 5 ml dilute hydrochloric acid in a boiling water bath for 5 minutes. Cool the solution and gently shake it with an organic solvent such as benzene. Remove the organic solvent layer and replace it with a similar amount of dilute ammonia. In the ammonical layer, a pinkish red colour develops. This is a C. glycoside test.

Therapeutic activity and Pharmaceutical Applications

A few examples are noted here

S. No.	Crude Drug	Chemical Constituents	Therapeutic activity and Pharmaceutical Applications
Anthracene glycosides:			
1.	Aloes	Barbaloin, aloe-emodin	Purgative
2.	Indian Senna	Sennosides A & B	Purgative
3.	Rhubarb	Rhein, Aloe-emodin	Purgative
Steroidal glycosides:			
4.	Digitalis	Purpurea glycoside A and B Lanatosides A and B	Cardiotonic
5.	Squill	Scillaren A and B	Cardiotonic
Saponin Glycosides:			
6.	Dioscorea	Diosgenin	Synthesis of medicinal steroids
7.	Ginseng	Ginsenosides	Stimulant, immunomdulator

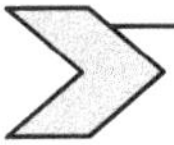

CHAPTER 5

Crude Drugs

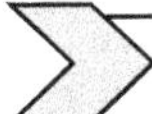

Laxatives

- *Laxatives* are a group of drugs that either accelerate fecal passage or decrease fecal consistency. They are used primarily to treat constipation.

  E.g.: Aloe, Castor oil, Ispaghula, Senna.

S. No.	Drug Name	Biological Source	Chemical Constituents	Therapeutic Efficacy
1.	Aloe	Aloe is the dried juice obtained from the leaves of various species of Aloe like *Aloe perryi* Baker, *Aloe vera* and *Aloe Africana* belonging to the family Liliaceae.	Aloin is the chief constituent of aloes it is the mixture of 3 isomers namely barbalion, iso-barbaloin, β-barbaloin. **Barbaloin**	• It is used as purgative. • It has also been suggested for relieving the stomach pain.
2.	Castor oil	It is a clear viscid fixed oil obtained from the seeds of *Ricinus communis* belonging to the family Euphorbiaceae.	It consists of glycerides of ricinoleic, isoricinoleic, stearic and dihydroxy-stearic acids. **Ricinoleic acid** $CH_3(CH_2)_5CH(OH)CH_2CH=CH(CH_2)_7COOH$	• It is used as cathartic. • In case of food poisoning the use of castor oil is used. • Used as Emollient. • Used in the preparations of paints, varnish, grease, polishes etc.

Table *Contd...*

S. No.	Drug Name	Biological Source	Chemical Constituents	Therapeutic Efficacy
3.	Senna	It is obtained from the dried leaflets of *Cassia acutifolia* and *Cassia angustifolia* belonging to the family Leguminosae.	It consists of Sennosides A, B, C and D which are present in the concentration of 2-3%. Senna also contains free chrysophanol and emodin, their glycosides and free aloe emodin, mucilage. Sennoside A Sennoside B	• Used as stimulant laxative. • Senna is stimulant cathartic and exerts its action by increasing the tone of the smooth muscles in the large intestine.

Cardiotonic

❖ Cardiotonics helps to increase the efficiency and improves the contraction of the heart muscle leading to improvement of blood flow to rest of the tissues in the body.

S. No.	Drug Name	Biological Source	Chemical Constituents	Therapeutic Efficacy
1.	Digitalis	It is obtained from the dried leaves of *Digitalis purpurea* and *Digitalis lanata* - family Scrophulariaceae.	❖ It contains primary and secondary glycosides and aglycone. ❖ Primary glycosides are Purpurea glycoside A and B. ❖ Secondary glycosides are Digitoxin, Digitoxigenin and Gitoxin. 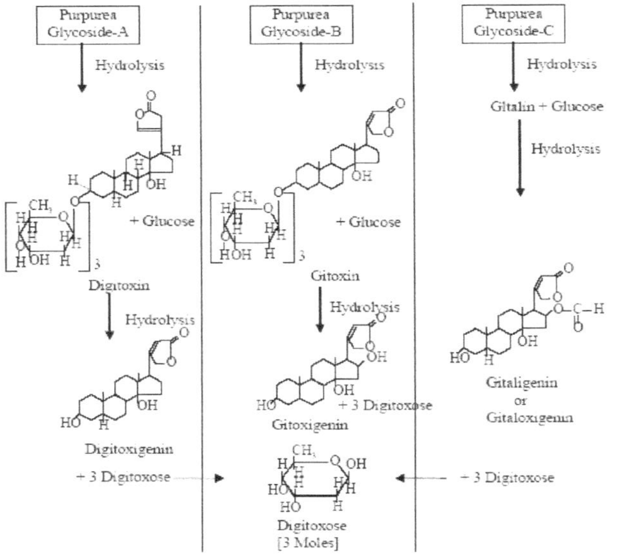	• It increases the activity of cardiac muscles. • It is useful in congestive heart failure, atrial flutter, atrial fibrillation.
2.	Arjuna	It is obtained from the bark of *Terminalia arjuna* - family Combretaceae.	❖ The bark is rich in tannins, terpenoids, saponins. ❖ Large amount of calcium salts and traces of aluminium and magnesium salts.	• It is used as diuretic and astringent. • It also used to decrease blood pressure. • It is used in various cardiac diseases.

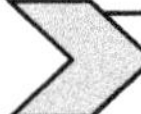 ## Carminatives and GI Regulators

❖ An agent that can cause expulsion of gas from the stomach or bowel is known as carminative.

S. No.	Drug name	Biological Source	Chemical Constituents	Therapeutic efficacy
1.	Coriander	It is obtained from the dried fruit of *Coriandrum sativum* belonging to the family Umbelliferae.	❖ The chief constituent is linalool (coriandrol) and α-pinene. (S)-(+)-Linalool (R)-(−)-Linalool ❖ Geraniol and borneol are present in traces.	• It is used as flavoring agent and carminative and also used for cooking purpose.
2.	Fennel	It is obtained from the dried ripened fruits of *Foeniculum vulgare* belonging - family Umbelliferae.	❖ The chief constituents are Anethole (50-60%), Fenchone (15-20%) ketone. **Anethole** **Fenchone** ❖ And it contains 20% of fixed oils and 20% of proteins.	• It is used as flavoring agent and carminative. It is used as respiratory stimulant and used in mouthwashes.
3.	Cardamom	It is obtained from the dried ripened fruits of *Elettaria cardamomum* - family Zingiberaceae.	❖ It contains volatile oils like terpinyl acetate and cineole. **Cineole**	• It is used as flavoring agent and also used as tincture in pharmacy.
4.	Ginger	It is obtained from the rhizomes of *Zingiber officinale* belonging to the family Zingiberaceae.	❖ The main constituents are three sesquiterpens bisabolene, zingiberene and zingiberol. **zingiberol**	• It is largely used as condiment and as an anti-emetic. • It is used as stimulant and carminative and also as flavoring agent.

Table *Contd...*

S. No.	Drug name	Biological Source	Chemical Constituents	Therapeutic efficacy
			❖ It also contains gingerol, oleoresin are zingirne and shogaol. ❖ Other constituents are starch and mucilage.	
5.	Clove	It is obtained from the dried flower bud of *Eugenia caryophyllus* - family Myrtaceae.	❖ The main volatile oil present in clove is Eugenol. **Eugenol** ❖ It also contains gallotannic acid, oleanolic acid, vanillin, eugenin and methyl amyl ketone.	● It is used as carminative and flavoring agent. ● Clove oil is used as antiseptic. ● It is commonly employed as a remedy for toothache and it acts like local anaesthetic.
6.	Black pepper	*Piper nigrum,* also known as black pepper is the member of *Piperaceae* family.	❖ It contains piperine, beta-carotene, lauric-acid, palmitic acid, and pepper phellandrene. Piperine	● It works as an analgesic, antipyretic and antioxidant. ● It utilizes as a rubefacient. ● It is also used as a preservative. ● It is used in the treatment of fever, colic, dysentery, piles and infections of worms.
7.	Asafoetida	Asafoetida is an oleo-gum-resin obtained by incising the living rhizomes and roots of *Ferula foetida* belonging to the family Umbelliferae	❖ It contains volatile oils, like isobutyl propanyl disulphate. The resin contains asaresinol ferulate and free ferulic acid. *trans* - Ferulic Acid Umbellic Acid Umbelliferone	● It is powerful nervine stimulant and used in nervous disorder of hysteria. Used in case of constipation.

Table *Contd...*

S. No.	Drug name	Biological Source	Chemical Constituents	Therapeutic efficacy
8.	Nutmeg	It is obtained from the arillus and seed coat of the dried ripe seed of *Myristica fragrans* - family Myristicaceae.	❖ Myristicin is the volatile oil present in it. It also contains Elemicin. Myristicin ❖ Protein and starch are the other constituents.	• It is used as flavoring agent and carminative and also used for diarrhea. • It produces narcotic and anaesthetic action on CNS and also produce halluginations.
9.	Cinnamon	It is obtained from the dried bark of *Cinnamomum zeylanicum* belonging to the family Lauraceae.	❖ It contains volatile oils, starch, phlobotannin mucilage and calcium oxalate. ❖ Cinnamon oil is the chief constituent it contains cinnamic aldehydes, eugenol and some hydrocarbons, ketones, esters and alcohols. **Eugenol**	• It is used as flavoring agent and carminative. • It is also used as mild astringent. The oil has powerful germicidal property.

▷ Astringents

❖ An agent contracting organic tissues, thereby lessening secretion includes drying and roughness in mouth.

S. No.	Drug Name	Biological Source	Chemical Constituents	Therapeutic Efficacy
1.	Myrobalan	It is obtained from dried mature big or immature small fruits of an Indian tree *Terminalia chebula* belonging to the family Combretaceae.	❖ It contains 30-40% of hydrolysable tannins. ❖ It contains fixed oil containing mainly esters of palmitic, oleic and linoleic acid.	• It is used as purgative. • Trifla is a popular formulation consisting of myrobalan, beleric and embelic fruits.

Table *Contd...*

S. No.	Drug Name	Biological Source	Chemical Constituents	Therapeutic Efficacy
2.	Black Catechu	Black catechu is a dried extract prepared by boiling the heart wood of *Acacia catechu* - family Leguminosae.	❖ It contains (+)-catechin and (+)-epicatechin, catechu tannic acid and flavonoid like quercetin. (+) Catechin (-)-Epicatechin (+) Epigallocatechin (-)-Epigallocatechin-3-gallate ❖ It also contains gummy material.	• It is used as astringent in diarrhea and for cleaning mouth and gums.
3.	Pale Catechu	It is an aqueous extract prepared from the leaves and young shoots of *Uncaria gambier* belonging to the family Rubiaceae.	❖ The drug mainly contains (+)-catechin (7-33%), catechutannic acid (22-50%). Other constituents are catechu red, quercitin and gambier fluorescin, a fluorescent substance. (+) Catechin (-)-Epicatechin (+) Epigallocatechin (-)-Epigallocatechin-3-gallate	• It is used as astringent, antidiarrhoeal and a local astringent in the form of lozenges. It is also used for tanning and dyeing

Drugs acting on Nervous System

S. No.	Drug Name	Biological Source	Chemical Constituents	Therapeutic Efficacy
1.	Hyoscyamus	It is obtained from the dried leaves of *Hyoscyamus niger* belonging to the family Solanaceae.	It contains about 1.5% of alkaloids of which the hyoscyamine and hyoscine are the active principles. **Hyoscine**	• It is used to relieve spasms of the urinary tract. • It often given with strong purgatives to prevent griping.

Table *Contd...*

S. No.	Drug Name	Biological Source	Chemical Constituents	Therapeutic Efficacy
2.	Belladona	It is obtained from the dried leaves and flowering tops of *Atropa belladona* - family Solanaceae.	It contains ¾ of hyoscyamine and remaining is atropine. Small quantities of pyridine and N-methyl pyrrolidine is also present. 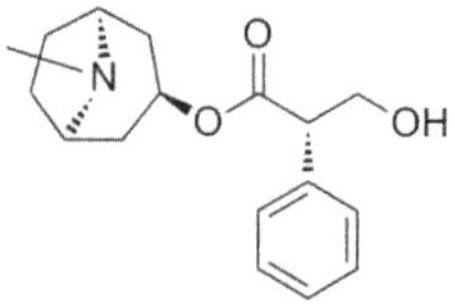 **Hyoscyamine**	• It acts as parasympathetic depressant. • It is used for control of spasms. • It is used to check excessive persipiration of patients suffering from TB.
3.	Ephedra	It is obtained from the entire plant of *Ephedra sinica* belonging to the family Gnetaceae.	It contains Ephedrine as major constituent. 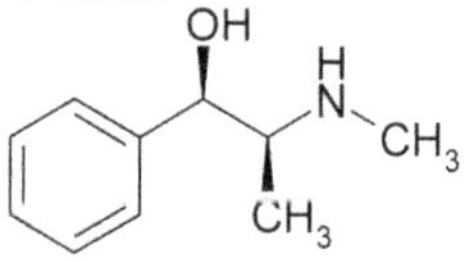 **Ephedrine** Pseudoephedrine is also present.	• It is used to relief asthma, rhinitis, whooping cough and hay fever. • It causes vasoconstriction.
4.	Opium	It is obtained by incising the unripened capsules of *Papaver somniferum* belonging to the family Papaveraceae.	It contains MT 25 alkaloids the most important alkaloids are morphine, 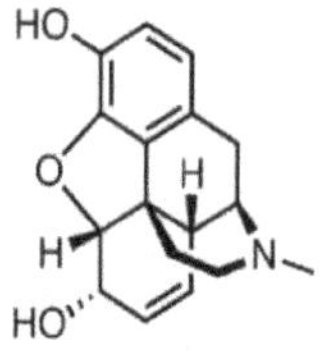 **Morphine** 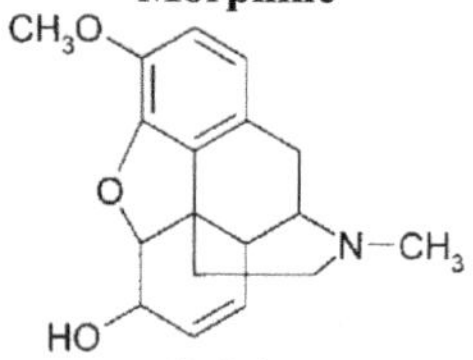 **Codeine** 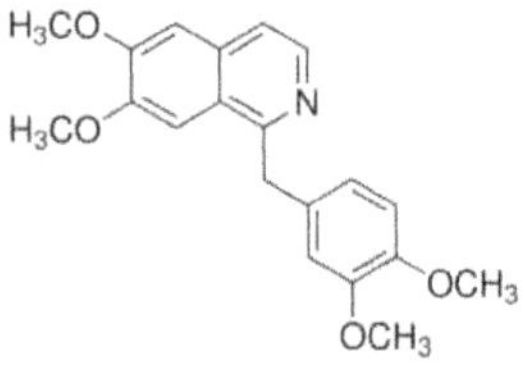 **Papaverine** codeine, narcotine, papaverine and thebaine.	• It is used as an analgesic, narcotic and hypnotic. • Codeine is used in cough syrups.

Table *Contd...*

S. No.	Drug Name	Biological Source	Chemical Constituents	Therapeutic Efficacy
5.	Tea leaves	It is obtained from *Thea sinensis* belonging to the family Theaceae.	It contains 1-5% of tannin and 10-24% of caffeine. It contains theobromine, theophylline, catechins, theoflavins, caffeine, polyphenol. 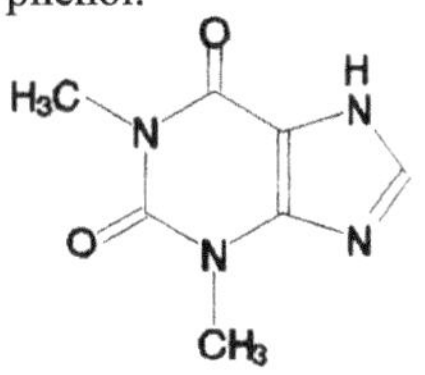 **Theophylline** 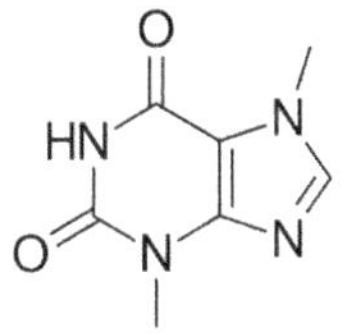 **Theobromine**	• It have stimulant effect on nervous system and heart and also as diuretic. • It is also used as astringent.
6.	Coffee seeds	It is the dried ripe seeds of *Coffea arabica* - the family Rubiaceae.	The main constituents - caffeine, tannins, fixed oils and proteins. 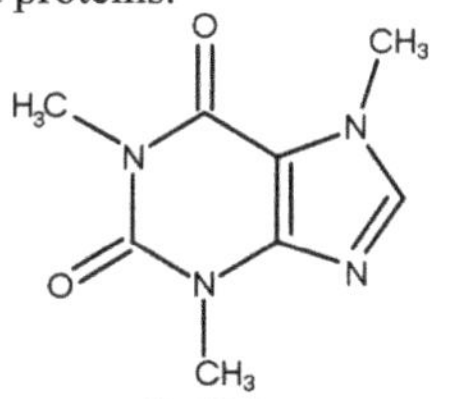 **Caffeine**	• Widely used as flavoring agent in ice creams, pastries etc., • It is used as stimulant, nervine and diuretic.
7.	Coca	It is obtained from the dried leaves of *Erythoylum coca* belonging to the family Erythroxylaceae.	It contains alkaloids in which cocaine, cinnamoylcocaina and α-or β-truilline are important. Hygrine, tropacocaine and cocatannic acid are present. 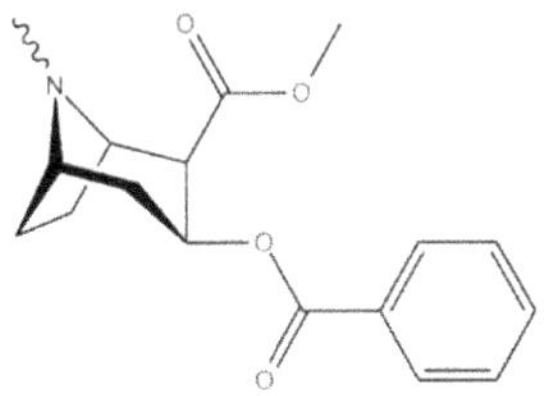 **Cocaine**	• CNS stimulant. • It is used in convalescence, to get rid of nausea, vomiting. • It is also local anesthetic action. • It is used as dental anesthesthetic .

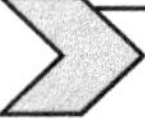

Antihypertensives

Antihypertensives are the category of medications to treat high blood.

S. No.	Drug Name	Biological source	Chemical constituents	Therapeutic efficacy
1.	Rauwolfia	It is the dried roots of *Rauwolfia serpentina* belongs to the family Apocynaceae.	The chief constituent is Reserpine Others- Serpentine, ajmaline, ajmalcine, rescinnamine, reserpinine, yohimbine, deserpidine Syrosingopine and serpentinine. **Reserpine**	• Antihypertensive drug which depletes catecholamines at nerve endings thereby lowers blood pressure. • Rescinnamine used to treat mental depression at higher doses. • Ajmalicine used in relief of obstruction of normal cerebral blood flow.

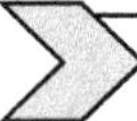

Antitussives

The opioid and nonopioid medicines that inhibit the cough reflex by acting on the central and peripheral nerve systems. Antitussives should not be taken with a productive cough since the cough reflex is required for clearing obstructive secretions from the upper respiratory tract.

S. No.	Drug name	Biological source	Chemical constituents	Therapeutic efficacy
1.	Vasaka	It consists of dried or fresh leaves of *Adhatoda Vasica* belonging to the family Acanthaceae.	It contains quinazoline derivatives of Vasicine, vasicinone, **Vasicine** adhatodic acid, adhatodine and vasicol.	• It is used as expectorant and bronchodilator. • In large doses it causes vomiting and diarrhoea. • It shows oxytocic property. It shows abortifacient activity.
2.	Tolu Balsam	It is the solid or semi-solid balsam obtained from trunk of trees *Myroxylon balsamum* - family Leguminosae.	It consists of 16 % free cinnamic acid. 8% free benzoic acid. It contains toluresinotannol, small quantities of vanillin and styrol. **Benzoic acid**	• It is used as an expectorant and flavouring agent. • It is also an antiseptic. • It is used in chewing gums and perfumery.

Table *Contd...*

S. No.	Drug name	Biological source	Chemical Constituents	Therapeutic efficacy
			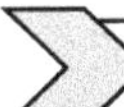 **Cinnamic acid**	

Antirheumatics

Antirheumatics are pain and stiffness relievers used to treat rheumatic disorders. Any medicine used to treat rheumatism is known as an antirheumatic.

S. No.	Drug name	Biological Source	Chemical constituents	Therapeutic efficacy
1.	Colchicum Seed	It consists of dried ripened seeds of *Colchicum luteum* and *Colchicum autumnale* belonging to the family Liliaceae	It consists of alkaloid – Colchicine is the chief constituent. It consists of demecolcine. It contains tropolone. **Colchicine**	• It is used in treatment of gout and rheumatism. • It possess antitumour activity. • It also brings polyploidy hence used in horticulture.

Antitumours

Antitumours are the drugs which inhibits the tumour growth.

S. No.	Drug name	Biological source	Chemical constituents	Therapeutic efficacy
1.	Vinca	It is the dried whole plant of *Catharanthus roseus* - family Apocynaceae.	It consists of vincristine and vinblastine. Vincristine acts by arresting the mitosis of cell at the stage of metaphase. **Vinblastine**	It acts as antineoplastic agent. It is used in hodgkins disease, lymphomas and also exhibits hypotensive and antidiabetic actions.

Table *Contd...*

S. No.	Drug name	Biological source	Chemical constituents	Therapeutic efficacy
			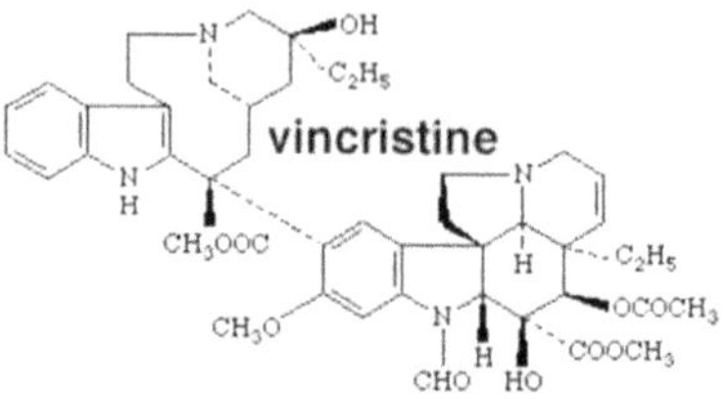 vincristine (structure)	
2.	Podophyllum	It consists of dried rhizomes and roots of *Podophyllum hexandrum* - family Berberidaceae.	It consists of podophyllin and etoposide. The active principle is podophyllotoxin. It consists of flavonoid-astragalin. Other constituents-Quercitin, Kaempferol, asiragalin. 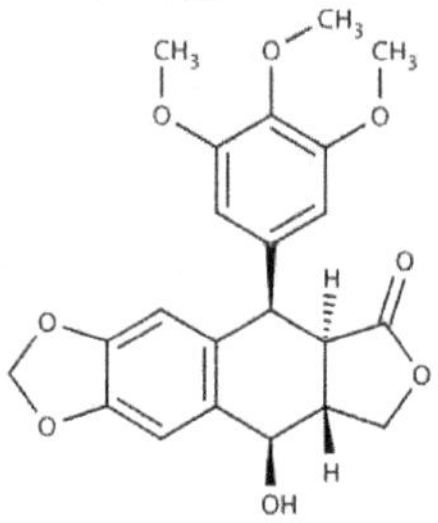 **Podophyllotoxin** (structure)	It is cytotoxic in action. It is also used in purgative and bitter tonic. It is used in semi-synthetic production of etoposide.

Antidiabetics

Antidiabetic pharmaceuticals are medications that assist diabetics manage their blood sugar levels (sugar diabetes).

S. No.	Drug Name	Biological source	Chemical constituents	Therapeutic efficacy
1.	Pterocarpus	It consists of dried juice of the plant *Pterocarpus marsupium* belonging to the family Leguminosae.	Kinotannic acid, Kinored, k-pyrocatechin, resin and gallic acid. Crystalline principle – santal, pterocarpan, and homopterocarpin.	It is used as powerful astringent. It is treatment diarrhoea and dysentery. It dyeing, tanning and printing. It also hypoglycemic action.
2.	Gymnema	Leaves of *Gymnema sylvestre* - family Asclepiadaceae.	It contains pentriacontane, hentriacontane, phytin. It contains Gymnemic acid as its chief constituent. 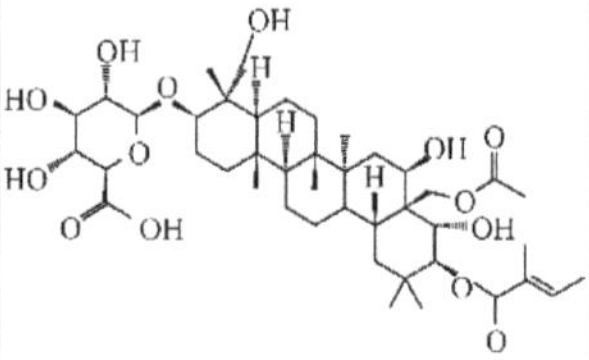 **Gymnemic acid** (structure)	It is used as antidiabetic, stimulant, laxative and diuretic. Dental plaque an caries are prevented.

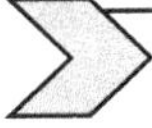 ## Diuretics

❖ A diuretic is any substance that promotes diuresis, the increased production of urine.

S. No.	Drug Name	Biological source	Chemical constituents	Therapeutic efficacy
1.	Gokhru	It is obtained from the dried ripened seeds of *Tribulus terrestris* - family Zygophyllaceae.	It consists chlorogenin, hecogenin and neotigo-genin. The other steroidal components - terestroside F, tribulosin, trillin etc.,	• It posses Anti-inflammatory, Anti-arthritic, diuretic, tonic, aphrodisiac properties.
2.	Punarnava	It is obtained from the fresh and dried of whole plant of *Boerhaavia diffusa* belonging to the family Nyctaginaceae.	It contains punarnavoside and boeravinones A, B, C, D, E. The root contains hypoxanthine-9-arabinofuranoside and boeravine, ursolic acid, β-sitosterol.	• It is used as antifibrinolytic, anti inflammatory, diuretic. • It is used to treat IUD menorrhagia. • The whole plant juice is used as blood purifier.

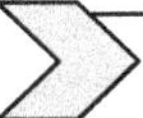 ## Antidysenterics

❖ *Dysentery* is an infection of the intestines that causes diarrhoea containing blood or mucus.

S. No.	Drug name	Biological source	Chemical Constituents	Therapeutic efficacy
1.	Ipecacuanha	It is obtained from the dried root or rhizome of *Cephaelis ipecacuanha or Cephaelis acuminata* - family Rubiaceae.	It contains emetine, cephaeline, psychotrine and psychotrine methyl ether.	• It is used as emetic and expectorant and diaphoretic and in the treatment of amoebic dysentery.

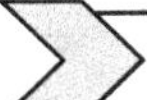 ## Antiseptics and Disinfectants

• Antiseptic is a substance that stops or slows down the growth of microorganisms.

• A disinfectant is a chemical substance or compound used to inactivate or destroy microorganisms on inert surfaces.

S. No.	Drug name	Biological source	Chemical constituents	Therapeutic efficacy
1.	Benzoin	It is a balsamic resin obtained from the incised stem of *Styrax benzoin* belonging to the family Styraceae.	Sumatra benzoin contains free balsamic acids, chiefly cinnamic and benzoin acids and ester derivatives, siaresinolic acid and sumaresionlic acid are also present. 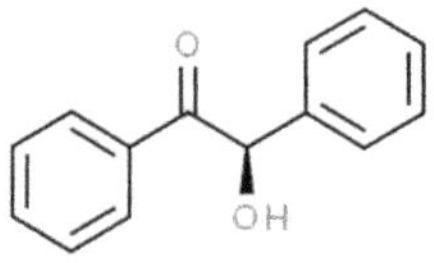 **Benzoin** 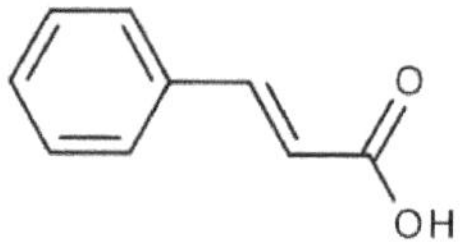 **Cinnamic acid** Siam benzoin consists of ester coniferyl benzoate, traces of vanillin and triterpene siaresinol is present.	• It possess antiseptic, expectorant and diuretic activity. • It is used as compound of henzoin tincture.
2.	Myrrh	It is an oleo-gum-resin obtained from the stem of *Commiphora molmol* belonging to the family Burseraceae.	It contains terpenes, esters, cuminic aldehyde and eugenol, commiphoric acid and phenolic compounds.	• It is used in incense and perfumes. • It is employed as stimulant and a stomachic. • It is used as astringent and disinfectant
3.	Neem	It is obtained from the plant *Azadirachta indica* belongingto the family Meliaceae.	Nimbidin is the chief constituent. Azadirachtin is found in seeds.	• It is used as astringent, antiseperiodic and also used in malaria. • Leaves are used to treat ulcers and eczema.
4.	Turmeric	It is obtained from the dried rhizomes of *Curcuma longa* belonging to the family Zingiberaceae.	It contains curcumin, volatile oils and sequiterpenes like turmerone and zingiberene.	• It is used as a colouring agent and condiment in curry. • It is used to treat gallstones, menstrual pains. • It is used as anti-inflammatory agent.

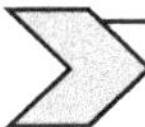

Anti-malarials

They are used to treat or prevent malaria.

S. No.	Drug name	Biological source	Chemical constituents	Therapeutic efficacy
1.	Cinchona	It is obtained from the dried stem or the bark or root of *Cinchona succirubra* belonging to the family Rubiaceae.	It contains quinine, quinidine, cinchonidine and chinhonine.	• It is used in the treatment of malaria. • It is used as bitter tonics and stomachics.
2.	Artemisia	It is obtained from the derived from the plant *Artemisia cina and A. maritina* belonging to the family Compositae.	Terpenoids, swsquiterpene, santonin, β-santonin, volatile oil: cineole, artemisin.	• Anthelmintic

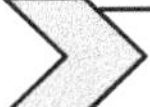

Oxytocin

➢ Oxytocin is a peptide hormone produced in the hypothalamus and released by the posterior pituitary.

S. No.	Drug Name	Biological source	Chemical constituents	Therapeutic efficacy
1.	Ergot	The biological source of ergot is dried sclerotinum of *Claviceps purpurea* belonging to the family clavicipitaceae.	Water soluble chemical constituents - Ergometrine and ergometrinine **Ergometrine** Water insoluble chemical constituents -Ergotamine, ergotaminine, ergosinine and ergosine. It is also composed of sterols - ergosterol and fungisterol.	• It is vasoconstrictor and abortifacient activity. • It is used in the treatment of migraine. • Partial synthesis of lysergic acid, which is a potent specific psychotomimetic. • It stimulates the tone of uterine muscles and prevent post-partum haemorrhage.

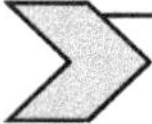 # Vitamins

Vitamins are any of a set of chemical substances that are required in small amounts in the diet because they cannot be produced by the body and are essential for normal growth and nutrition.

S. No.	Drug name	Biological source	Chemical constituents	Therapeutic efficacy
1.	Shark Liver oil	It is the fixed oil obtained from fresh and preserved livers of *Hypoprion brevirostris* and *Galeorhinus zyopterus*.	It contains vitamin A. Other constituents are glycerides of the saturated and unsaturated fatty acids along with alkyl glycerol. It contains squalene and omega-3-fattyacids. **Vitamin A**	• It is used in the defieciency of Vitamin A. • It is also known as antixeropthalmic factor. • It is used in burn and sunburn ointments.
2.	Cod Liver Oil	It is processed from fresh liver of cod fish, *Gadus morrhua* belonging to the family Gadidae	The oil contains Vitamin A & D. It contains glyceryl esters of oleic, linoleic, gadoleic, myristic, palmitic and other acids. It contains 7% eicosapentaenoic acid and 7% docesahexanoic acid.	• It is nutritive. • Used in the treatement of rickets and TB.

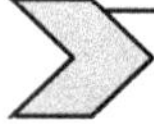 # Enzymes

An enzyme is a protein which is a catalyst in living organisms controls the chemical reactions.

S. No.	Drug name	Biological source	Chemical constituents	Therapeutic efficacy
1.	Papaya	It contains papain. Papain is a proteolytic enzyme obtained from latex of unripened fruits of *Carica papaya* belonging to the family Caricaceae.	It contains mixture of papain and chymopapain. It is a proteolytic enzymes act on polypeptides and amides.	• It is used in clarification of beverages and as a meat tenderizer. • It is used as degumming of silk fibrics in textile industry. • It is used in leather industry for removing hair of skins. • It is used as an anti-inflammatory agent. It relieves the symptoms of episiotomy.

Table *Contd...*

S. No.	Drug name	Biological source	Chemical constituents	Therapeutic efficacy
2.	Diastase	It is an amylolytic substance present in saliva or found in the digestive tracts of animals. It is also present in barley grains during germination.	It catalyses the hydrolysis of 1,4-glycosidic linkage of polysaccharides like starch and glycogen.	• It is used as digestant. It is used in the production of predigested starchy foods and conversion of starch to fermentable sugars.
3.	Pancreatin	It is the preparation extracted from pancreas of animals like hog -Sus scrofa belonging to the family Suidae.	It contains mainly amylase, lipase and protease.	• It is used in pancreatic deficiency like pancreatitis and also in fibrocytic diseases of pancreas. • It is also used for predigested food. • It is employed as digestive aid for converting starch into dextrin and sugar, proteins into proteases and fats into glycerol and fatty acids.
4.	Yeast	Yeasts are chemoorganotrophs, meaning they get their energy from organic chemicals rather than sunlight. Saccharomyces cerevisiae is a single-celled organism that requires food, temperature, and moisture to grow. Brewer's yeast, a wet yeast used largely in beer production, and baker's yeast, a leavening agent, are the two forms of yeast available.	Catalase is an enzyme found in yeast that works as a catalyst in the breakdown of hydrogen peroxide into oxygen and water ($2H_2O_2$ $2H_2O + O_2$).	• It is used brewing beer. • Used in making chocolates. • Used to prevent hair loss. • It moisturizes skin. • It is a source of protein.

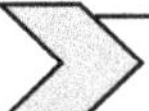

Pharmaceutical Aids

Pharmaceutical aids and necessities are **the agents important in Preparations for preservation, binding etc.,**

S. No.	Drug Name	Biological source	Chemical constituents	Therapeutic efficacy
1.	Kaolin	It is a purified native hydrated aluminium silicate free from gritty particles. It is obtained by powdering the native kaolin.	It types of kaolin are 1. Heavy Kaolin: contains hydrated aluminium silicate 2. Light kaolin: identical to heavy kaolin. 3. Natural light kaolin: native hydrated aluminium silicate free from gritty particles	• It is used as an adsorbent. • Used in the treatment of enteritis, dysentery and food poisoning. • It is applied externally as dusting powder.
2.	Lanolin	Hydrous wool fat is a purified fat like substance obtained from wool of the sheep Ovis aries belonging to the family Bovidae.	It contains mainly esters of cholesterol and isocholesterol with carnaubic, oleic, myristic, palmitic, lignoceric and lanopalmitic acids.	• It is used as water absorbale ointment base. It is the common ingredient and base for several water soluble creams and cosmetic preparations. It also can be allergic.
3.	Beeswax	It is the purified wax obtained from honey comb of the bees Apis mellifica belongs to the family Apidae.	It contains esters of straight chain monohydric alcohols. It contains myricin, free cerotic acid, melissic acid and cerolein.	• It is used in the preparation of ointments, plasters and polishes. • Used in ointment for hardening purpose. • Used in cosmetics in the preparations of lipsticks and face creams. • It is an ingredient present in Paraffin ointment IP.
4.	Acacia	It is the dried gummy exudation obtained from stems and leaves of *Acacia arabica* belonging to the family Leguminosae.	It consists of arabin, is a complex mixture of calcium, magnesium and potassium salts of Arabic acid. Arabic acid on hydrolysis gives L-arabinose. L-rhamnose, D-galactose and D-glucuronic acid.	• It is used as a demulcent. • Used in haemolysis. • It is used in suspending agent. • Good emulsifying agent. • Used in the preparation of lozenge, compressed pills and microencapsulation of drugs.

Table *Contd...*

S. No.	Drug Name	Biological source	Chemical constituents	Therapeutic efficacy
5.	Tragacanth	It is a dried gummy exudation obtained by incision from stems and branches of *Astragalus gummifer* belonging to the family Leguminosae.	It contains two fractions. Water soluble fraction – Tragacanthin. Water insoluble fraction – Bassorin. It contains 15% of methoxy group because of it swells in water.	• Used as a demulcent and emollient in cosmetics. • It is used as thickening, suspending and emulsifying agent. • Used as binding agent in tablets • It is used as an adhesive. • Used in spermicidal jellies.
6.	Sodium alginate	It is the sodium salt of alginic acid. Alginic acid is a polyuronic acid composed of reduced mannuronic acid and glucuronic acid.	Alginic acid is a linear co-polymer. It contains d-mannopyranosyluronic acid linked with L-glucopyranosyluronic acids units.	• Used in the preparation of paste, creams, thickening and stabilizing emusions. • It is a good suspending agent. • Used as binding and disintegrating agent. • Used in textile industry.
7.	Agar	It is dried gelationous substance obtained from *Gelidium amansii* belonging to the family Gelidaceae.	It contains two different polysaccharides agarose and agaropectin. Agarose is responsible for gel strength and Agaropectin is responsible for viscosity of agar solution.	• It is used in emulsifying agent and bulk laxative. • Used in the preparation of jellies. • Used m bacteriological culture medium.
8.	Guar gum	It is the powder of endosperm of seeds of *Cyamopsis tetragonolobus* belonging to the family Leguminosae.	It contains water soluble portion known as guaran. Upon hydrolysis guaran gives 65% galactose and 35% mannose. It also contains water insoluble portions. It contains 5-7% of proteins.	• Used as a protective colloid. • It is used as binding and disintegrating agent, • It is appetite depressant and peptic ulcer therapy. • It is good emulsifying agent. • Used in manufacture of paper, printing and polishing. • Used in food and cosmetic industries

Table Contd...

S. No.	Drug name	Biological source	Chemical constituents	Therapeutic efficacy
9.	Gelatin	It is a protein extracted by partial hydrolysis of animal collagenous tissue like skins, tendons, ligaments and bones in a boiling water.	It contains different aminoacids which major one is lysine, an essential aminoacid but it doesnot contain tryptophan. It is composed of Gluten protein.	• It is used in manufacture of hard and flexible capsule shells. • Used in preparation of pessaries, pastes, pastilles and suppositories. • It is used as haemostatic. • It is employed in microencapsulation of drugs. • Used in perfumes, flavours and used as vehicle in certain injections. • It is used in bacteriological culture media.

Miscellaneous

S. No.	Drug name	Biological source	Chemical constituents	Therapeutic efficacy
1.	Squill	It consist of sliced and dried scaly leaves from the bulbs of *Urginea maritima* belonging to the family Liliaceae. (Eurpeon Squill). It consists of dried slices of bulb of *Urginea indica* belonging to the family Liliaceae. (Indian Squill)	It consists of Scillaren A and B. Scillaren A upon hydrolysis by the enzyme scillarenase gives proscillaridin A and upon acid hydrolysis Scillaridin A. Scillaren B upon enzyme hydrolysis gives proscillaridin B and on acid hydrolysis gives Scillaridin B.	• It is cardiotonic and expectorant. • It is diuretic in small doses. • It also possess anti-cancer activity.

Table Contd...

S. No.	Drug name	Biological source	Chemical constituents	Therapeutic efficacy
2.	Galls	It is the pathological out growth formed on young twigs of *Quircus infectoria* belonging to the family Fagaceae.	It contains 50-70% of tannic acid. Upon hydrolysis it gives gallic acid and glucose. It is incompatible with alkaloids, gelatin, albumin and iron salts	• Used as an astringent for mucous membrane of mouth and throat. • It is effective in treatment of piles. • It is an antidote for poisoning of alkaloids, he
3.	Ashwagandha	It consists of dried roots and stem bases of *Withania somnifera* belonging to the family Solanaceae.	Withanine is the main constituent present in it. Somniferine, somnine, somniferinine, withananine, tropine, pseudotropine, pseudowithanine, anaferine and anahydrine. It contains steroidal lactones called Withanolides.	• It is sedative and hypnotive. • It is used in hypotensive, respiratory stimulant. • It is an immune-modulatory agent. • It posess antistress activity. • It is used in the treatment of rheumatism, gout, hypertension, nervine and skin disease. • The leaf extract acts against Ranikhet virus.
4.	Tulsi	It consists of fresh and dried leaves of *Ocimum sanctum* belonging to the family Lamiaceae.	It contains 70% eugenol. Carvacrol and eugenol-methyl-ether. It contains caryophyllin. It contains traces of maleic, citric and tartaric acid.	• It is used as antibacterial and
5.	Guggul	It is the oleo-gum-resin obtained by making deep decisions at the basal part of stem bark of *Commiphora weightii* belonging to the family Burseraceae	It contains Guggulosterone-s and guggulosterol I. It contains Guggulosterone-Z, E-guggulosterone and the 3 new sterols – guggulosterol I, II and III.	• It is used as anti-inflammatory, anti-rheumatic and hypo-cholesteremic drug. • It lowers low density lipoproteins. • It is antihyperlipidaemic product.

> **CHAPTER 6**

Plant Fibres

Fibre ultimate is defined as "one of the component botanical cells within which leaf and bast fibers can be distinguished." A fibre is defined as "a unit of matter defined by flexibility, fineness, and a higher amount of length to thickness," while a fibre is defined as "a unit of matter defined by flexibility, fineness, and a higher amount of length to thickness." And over 10,000 years have passed since these found naturally cellulosic fibres were first used. Cellulosics were utilised for fabrics in the Middle East and Asia around 8,000 B.C. Clothing is made of flax fibres, for example, dates back to roughly 3000 B.C., and the Babylonians utilised flax fibre for funerary purposes circa 650 B.C. Plant fibres. Surgical dressings are important in medical and pharmaceutical field.

Dressing makes a direct contact with wound while bandage holds the dressing in place. Dressings are continuously used during first aid and nursing to ensure healing, to stop tissue damage and mechanical hazards. An ideal Wound dressing should be sterile, breathable and conducive for a moist healing environment. The quality of surgical dressings depends on the type of the fibre used to prepare the dressing. Plant fibres include epidermal trichomes (cotton), phloem or bast fibres (jute), and pericyclic fibres (flax, hemp), while fibres of animal origin include wool and silk.

The selected fibres have been divided into three primary class categories based on their morphological structure: (a) bast fibres, which are formed from plant stems, (b) leaf fibres, which are produced from plant leaves, and (c) seed hair fibres, which will contain fruit fibres for convenience.

The mechanical properties of fibres are influenced by physical qualities such as structure, regularity or irregularities along across the fibres main axis, crystalline packed order, nebulous content, and chemical composition. Plant fibres, in fact, are composites in nature, with cellulose microfibrils acting as reinforcement in a lignin and hemicellulose matrix. The rule of mixtures can be used to anticipate the finding of mechanical properties (ROM). For example, the rigidity or modulus of the plant fibres cell wall all along fibres axis is calculated using the equation.

$$E_f = Vc\ EcCos^2\theta + Vnc\ Enc$$

Where,

E_f = Effective Modulus of the Fibre

E_c and E_{nc} = The elastic moduli of the crystalline and non-crystalline regions

V_c and V_{nc} = The volume fractions of crystalline and non-crystalline regions and

θ = Microfibril angle.

A few examples of plant fibres are stated below:

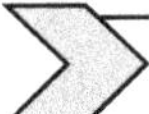 ## Cotton

Biological source

It contains of the hairs and epidermal trichomes of the seeds of *Gossypium barbadense* and other species of *Gossypium* belonging to the family Malvaceae.

Large scale production

The largest amount of cotton comes from United States of America India and Egypt. India stands in the second largest place in production of cotton.

Constituents

Raw cotton contains cellulose 91%, wax, oil and fat 0.4%, protoplasm, other cell constituents 0.6%, ash 0.2% and moisture 7.8%.

Preparation Cotton for surgical use

- Absorbent cotton wool is made from cotton waste i.e., hairs which are rejected by certain machinery during preparation of cotton for spinning (comber waste).

- Impurities are first removed and the cotton hair is then boiled with a 5% solution of caustic soda for about 15 hours at a pressure 1 to 3 atmospheres.

- After thorough washing with water, it is bleached by immersion for 10 to 18 hours in a 5% of chlorinated lime solution, washing with water and transferring to very dilute HCl acid for about 4hours.

- Next it is washed with water and treated with dil. HCl for 20 minutes, washed again, dried, loosened machinery and carded a kind of mechanical process or further separated by a current of hot air to make a fleecy, absorbent wool.

- This treatment removes the cuticle which consists of fatty matter composed of wax with stearic and palmitic acid.

Uses

Cotton is used as a filtering medium, and as the chief constituent of may surgical dressings and as a insulating material.

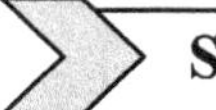

Silk

Biological source

Silk is a fiber made from the threads from the cocoons spun by the larvae of certain moths, the finest silk 'Mulberry Silk' is obtained from the larvae of Bombyx mori belonging to the family Bombycidae.

Constituents

Silk consists protein fibroin, coated externally by another protein, sericin or silk-gum, the proteins of silk contain C, H, O and N.

Uses

It is pharmaceutically for making ligatures, oiled silk and certain type of sieve.

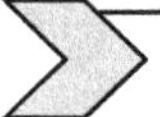

Wool

Biological source

It consists of the hairs from the fleece of the sheep, *Ovis aries* belonging to the family Bovidae.

Preparation

The hairs which forms fleece were removed from sheep at shearing time and thoroughly cleansed with soap or alkali carbonates to remove dirt and wool-grease. Wool is subjected for bleaching by treating with Sulphur dioxide or hydrogen peroxide. Then it is thoroughly washed and dried by hot air. The wool grease, after careful purification, forms the valuable wax known as wool-fat or lanolin.

Constituents

Wool consists almost entirely of keratin, and also C, H, O, N and S as elements.

It even contains nitrogen, Sulphur and 10-16 % moisture.

Uses

Wool is pharmaceutically used as a filtering and straining medium and for the manufacturing such materials as flannel, domette and crepe bandages.

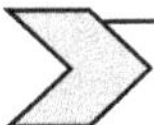 **Regenerated Fibers**

The raw sources for this fabric are natural materials including wood, bamboo, and cotton linters. Viscose rayon is manufactured as continuous filament and staple fibres, with staple fibres accounting for 90% of viscose rayon production. Due to high labour costs and rigorous environmental regulations, viscose rayon production has relocated from Europe, the United States, and other industrialised countries to the Asia–Pacific area since the twenty-first century.

Regenerated fibre is made by dissolving plant fibre cellulosic area in chemicals. Since it consists of cellulose like cotton and hemp hence called "regenerated cellulose fibre."

E.g.: Viscose, rayon, acetate, triacetate, modal, Tencel, and Lyocell.

Some of the regenerated cellulosic fibres are:

1. **Viscose Rayon Fiber**

   Silk fibre, pleasant feel, and drape features are all superb aesthetic properties of viscose fabric. Due to the presence of cellulose backbone in their structure, viscose has qualities similar to cotton or other cellulosic fibres. When compared to cotton, viscose has a higher moisture absorption. Other advantages of viscose fibres are breathability, softness, comfort, and ease of dyeing with vibrant colours.

   Dry strength and abrasion resistance are both good for viscose rayon. It is, nevertheless, prone to wrinkle formation because to its low resilience. It has a lower heat resistance than cotton. Viscose is commonly blended with a variety of other fibres to reduce cost or increase qualities like as shine, softness, absorbency, and comfort. Viscose rayon has a limited resistance to acids and alkalis, although it is resistant to bleaching chemicals and organic solvents.

2. **Bamboo Viscose Fiber**

   Bamboo viscose is a 100 percent cellulosic fabric derived from natural resources that may decompose fully in soil with the help of microorganisms and sunlight, with no negative environmental consequences. Because of the countless microlevel gaps and holes in its cross-section, bamboo viscose fibre is extremely breathable and cool. The moisture absorption and ventilation qualities of this fibre are excellent.

3. **Cellulose Acetate Fiber**

   This fibre is smoother than viscose as well as other textile fibres and has a good shine. Cellulose acetate offers excellent handling and comfort features (soft, smooth, dry, crisp, and robust) (breathes, wicks, dries quickly, and no static cling). Fabrics composed of cellulose acetate have excellent handling qualities and can be dyed to a variety of bright, soft, and appealing colours.

4. Lyocell Fibre

It degrades fully in the body. It has a high moisture absorption capacity. Lyocell fibre, unlike viscose, has excellent strength in both wet and dry circumstances. Other fibres, including as linen, wool, and cotton, can readily be combined with this fibre. Lyocell fibre fibrillates when it is abraded while wet, resulting in the development of surface fibrils. These surface fibrils are still linked to the fibres, but they peel away from the fibre surface, creating an appealing look.

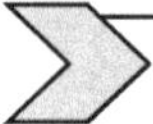

Sutures and Ligatures

Surgical ligatures and sutures are threads or strings specially prepared and strings specially prepared and sterilised for use in surgery. Numerous materials have been used like intestinal tissues, tendons of a large assortment of animals and birds, thread spun from vegetable fibres, hairs of humans, horse and camel, synthetic and metallic threads.

The most essential properties of ligatures and sutures are the following:

- It must be sterile.
- It should be with adequate strength.
- It should be fine guage.
- If absorbable the approximate time of absorption should be known.

Natural Suture Materials

A few examples of natural suture materials are Silk, Catgut.

Silk

Biological Source

The fibres are from the cocoons by the larvae *Bombyx mori* Linn., belonging to family Bombycidae.

Geographical Source

It is native to northern China and Persia presently known as Iran. Occurrence is from China, France, Iran, Italy, Japan, and India.

Preparation

The silkworms eat mulberry leaves day and night and their growth will be rapid. During the time of moult their head color changes darker. For a period of one month, full development takes place which attains a size of 9 cm length and 10 mm thick. The development results in tight and covers itself with a silky cocoon called spinning which takes place for almost 3 days. The larvae changes into chrysalides. The cocoons were thrown into boiling water which kills silkworms and also makes the cocoons easier to unravel. The unraveled cocoons were kept in hike warm water to remove the gum. Some amount of cocoons are retained and allowed to come out for fertilization. The females silkworms lays nearly 500 eggs and these were stored for further requirement.

Description

Color: Yellow

Size: 5-25 microns in diameter and 1200 meter in length

Appearance: Fine, solid, smooth to touch

Solubility: Soluble in cuoxam, dil. Sulphuric acid.

It is hygroscopic in nature and has good elasticity and tensile strength.

Chemical Constituents

It contains a protein called as fibrion. It is soluble in warm water and upon hydrolysis it yields amino acids viz., glycine and alanine.

Uses

It is used in the preparation of sutures, sieves, and ligatures. The 'stiff silkworm' is used in the traditional Chinese medicine.

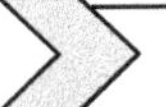 **Catgut**

This is the most widely used absorbable suture and ligature material. Catgut or violin gut is prepared from the intestine of the sheep. The name is said to be derived from the word 'kitgut'. Gut sutures have been used for hundreds of years and it is said that Rhazes of Baghdad used hard strings for surgical suturing over a thousand years ago.

When the sheep are slaughtered, the intestines are roughly deprived of their contents and placed in cold storage or packed in brine for transport. About the first 7-5m of the intestine is selected for surgical gut preparation.

Steps involved in the preparation of catgut are:
- Selection and washing
- Splitting the Casings
- Removal of unwanted layers
- Orientation of fibres
- Hardening
- Spinning
- Drying

- Finishing
- Gauging
- Sterilization
- Difficulties
- The heat process
- The irradiation process

All the catgut for surgical use in the UK is subjected to sterility tests under the Therapeutic Substances Act.

CHAPTER 7

Traditional System of Medicine

The Indian system of medicine is deeply ingrained in our cultural past and serves a sizable portion of our population's Medicare needs. Most of these methods rely on herbs. Due to the severe cumulative and irreversible side effects of many contemporary medications, the market has recently shifted in favour of herbal remedies.

Ayurveda, unani, siddha, yoga, and naturopathy are examples of Indian medical systems that have developed over time. One of the earliest collections of human knowledge is the Rigveda.

Ayurveda

* The words "ayur" and "veda," which together imply "life" and "knowledge or science," respectively, are the roots of the name "ayurveda," or "science of life."
* Ayurveda developed around 5000 years ago in the remote Himalayas, perhaps from the profound knowledge of prophets or Rishis who had attained spiritual enlightenment.
* The foundation of Ayurveda is the connection of the body, mind, and spirit.
* According to ayurveda, the universe's items, including the human body, are made up of five fundamental substances known as "Panchamahabhutas": earth, water, fire, air, and vacuum.
* The nutrition of the body matrix, or the food it consumes, which is made up of five elements, determines its growth and development.

Basic Principles of Ayurveda

The universe, according to traditional Indian philosophy, is made up of five fundamental substances known as panchabhutas: prithvi (earth), jal (water), teja (fire), vayu (air), and akash (space). These bhutas are the source of everything in the universe, including food and human bodies. Therefore, there is a basic harmony between the macrocosm (the universe) and the microcosm (the individual). The human body with the PanchaBhuta theory: The state of the human body is one of constant flux or dynamic balance. The doshas, dhatus, and malas in the human body are the pancha bhutas' physical representations.

In the body, there are three doshas. They are pitta, kapha, and vata. These three doshas have direct counterparts, called tridoshas. However, the representatives of vata are those that cause movement and sensation in a single cell or throughout the entire body; this explains all of the biological phenomena that are governed by the activities of the central and autonomous nerve systems. The representatives of pitta include the elements involved in digestion, metabolism, tissue growth, heat production, blood pigmentation, endocrine gland activity, and energy. The representatives of kapha are the elements that support the limbs' rigidity, nourish the sense organs, and support the stomach and joints. Each dosha predominates in certain specific body parts, including the chest.

Each of the dhatus, which make up the body's basic structure and constitute its elements, serves a specific purpose. The seven dhatus are: rakta (haemoglobin part of the blood), rakta (food juices), mamsa (muscular tissue), medas (fat tissue), asthi (bone tissue), majja (bone marrow), and shukra (semen).

The by-products of the dhatus are called malas. After the digestive process is complete, the body uses some of the malas and excretes the rest as waste. When these are gone, the supporting role they were performing while they were still inside the body is complete. Useful substances kept by the body are referred to as prasad (useful matter), whilst those expelled are referred to as malas (waste matter). The three main malas are sweda, shakrit, and mutra (urine) (perspira-tion). For the body to stay healthy, the doshas, dhatus, and malas must be in perfect equilibrium. Any unbalance between these components leads to sickness and poor health.

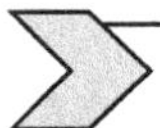 **Siddha**

One of India's most ancient medical systems is the Siddha system. The word "Siddha" implies success, and "Siddhars" were holy individuals who used Yoga to advance medicine. The Siddha system is practised in India's Tamil-speaking regions, and its literature is written in Tamil. After its well-known exponent Sage Agasthya, this system is often referred to as the Agasthyar system.

This system's core and applied ideas and tenets closely resemble those of ayurveda. The human body is a duplicate of the universe, according to this theory.

This theory, like ayurveda, holds that all things in the cosmos, including the human body, are made of five elements: earth, water, fire, air, and sky.

All five elements are present in food, beverages, and medications that the human body consumes.

Similar to ayurveda, this approach sees the body as a combination of three humours, seven fundamental tissues, and bodily fluids like faeces, urine, and sweat. Food is regarded as the fundamental component of the organism, from which humours, body tissues, and waste products are produced. A healthy body is one in which the humours are in balance, and one in which their distribution or imbalance results in illness or disease.

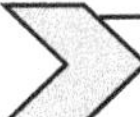

Unani

Greece is where the Unani medical system first emerged. Hippocrates' teachings form the foundation of the unani medical school's theoretical framework. By incorporating the best practises from modern traditional medical systems in Egypt, Syria, Iraq, Persia, India, China, and other middle-eastern and fast-eastern nations, unani medicine was enriched.

The Arabs introduced the unani medical technique to India. Unani intellectuals and doctors fled to India as the Mongols destroyed cities in Persia and Central Asia. The Unani system quickly established itself in Indian culture.

According to unani, the human body is made up of seven parts: afal (functions), aklath (humours), anza (organs), arawh (spirits), quo (faculties), and arkan (elements), each of which is closely related to a person's condition of health. Before making a diagnosis and recommending a course of therapy, a doctor takes all of these things into account.

It has established six crucial prerequisites for illness prevention. These necessities, often referred to as "Asbabe-Sita-Zarooriya," include air, food, and liquids, as well as physical motion and reaction, sleep and wakefulness, excretion, and retention. The Unani method places a strong emphasis on both preserving a healthy natural balance and preventing contamination of the water, food, and air.

In the Unani medical system, treatment entails the use of a single medicine, failing which a compound preparation may be used. The numerous therapies include "llajinit-dawa" (pharmacotherapy), "llajinit-ghiza" (diet therapy), and "llajbit-tadbeer" (regime therapy) (surgery). Physicians employ naturally occurring drugs, primarily herbs, in pharmacotherapy. The benefit of using naturally occurring medications is that their adverse effects are either comparable to or lower than those associated with the allopathic medical system.

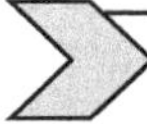 # Homeopathy

In accordance with the adage "Likes are treated by likes," Dr. Samuel Christian Friedrich Hahnemann (1755–1843), a German physician, chemist, and pharmacist, established the specialised treatment approach known as homoeopathy.

Pathos is the word for therapy, and homoios implies like (alike). Homoeopathy, then, is a technique of healing by the administration of medicines with the ability to cause similar pain (diseases) in healthy people. Dr. Hahnemann held the opinion that symptoms are not a physical representation of the sickness but rather the body's internal struggle to overcome it. Since the time of Hippocrates, the father of medicine, this law of similarity has been applied to the treatment of illnesses. But it was Dr Hahnemann who developed it in to a complete system of therapeutics enunciating the law and its application in 1810.

Fundamental Principles of Homoeopathy

Every science is guided by a set of fundamental principles. As a science of medicine, homoeopathy has its own philosophy, and its therapies are founded on some fundamental ideas that are quite separate from those of other medical schools. Hahnemann covered these key ideas in several chapters of his philosophy and medicine.

They are as follows:
1. Law of Similia.
2. Law of Simplex.
3. Law of minimum.
4. Drug proving.
5. Drug dynamization or potentization.
6. Vital force.
7. Acute and Chronic Diseases.
8. Individualization.
9. Direction of cure.

Law of similia

Simillia Similibus Curentur, which translates to "Let likes be treated by likes," is the foundational therapeutic principle of homoeopathy. In this form of medicine, the treatment for a patient with a sickness is designed to cause the same diseases in a healthy person as it does in the patient with the disease. In order to pick and administer Simillimum with confidence to treat, it is necessary to match the symptoms of the ill person with the pathophysiology of the medicine. Simillimum is one of the medicines that is most simila

Law of simple

At a time, simple and isolated medications should be administered. As a result, drugs are tested on healthy people alone and in pure form, without the addition of any other ingredient.

Law of minimum

Due to illness hypersensitivity, medications are always given in small doses, and their actions are always directed toward normal tissue due to altered tissue receptivity. The only purpose of the medications is to cause a response in the body. They have physiological actions that result in undesirable side effects and organic damage when administered in high quantities. The smallest amount of medication is necessary to approach the ailment because it has a very subtle nature. Only by utilising the smallest amount of medicine is it possible to anticipate the therapeutic activity of a drug without any unintended aggravation.

Drug proving

Knowing a drug's curative potential is necessary before using it for therapeutic purposes. When used on a healthy person, a drug's ability to cause disease symptoms is what makes it have curative power. The pathophysiology of a medicine can be used to determine its curative potential, which is then confirmed by testing the drug alone on healthy humans. The only accurate record of a drug's curative abilities is provided by this.

Drug dynamization or potentization

Disease is a disruption or departure from the dynamic life force's regular, harmonious flow. Today's drugs used to treat illnesses should also have a dynamic activity to counteract the dynamic disruption of life force. As a result, the medications are dynamized or potentized, releasing the dormant dynamic curative force. This dynamization is carried out using either the Trituration (for insoluble compounds) or Succession processes (in case of soluble substances).

Preparation of potencies

Three different scales, including decimal, centesimal, and millesimal, can be used to prepare the potency.

Vital force

Disease is nothing more than an unbalanced vital force flow that results in aberrant sensations and functions (symptoms and signs). The disorganised vital energy must be returned to normal in order to restore health. The vital force that powers health and disease are two different quantitative states of the same thing, and this is where treatment comes into play. Spiritual, autocratic, automatic, dynamic, stupid, and instinctual are some of the traits of vital force.

Acute and chronic diseases

According to the way the diseases start, progress, and end, they are divided into these categories.

Individualization

No two people in the world are same, thus diseases that affect people can never be the same assuming the distinctive individual picture in each diseased person. As a result, prescribing medications based solely on a disease's name is impossible because each disease case must be treated on an individual basis.

Direction of cure

According to Dr. Hering, "the treatment occurs within outward from above to lower, and the symptoms vanish in the opposite of their appearance." If the direction is the opposite of what is claimed, then suppression rather than treatment has taken place.

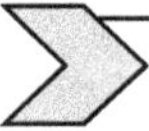 ## Ayurvedic Preparations

Pharmaceutical dosage forms prepared from the parts of plants like leaves, roots, rhizomes, wood, bark, fruits, seeds, tubers, rhizomes, corns, flowers and flowering buds used to combat diseases, are termed as herbal preparations.

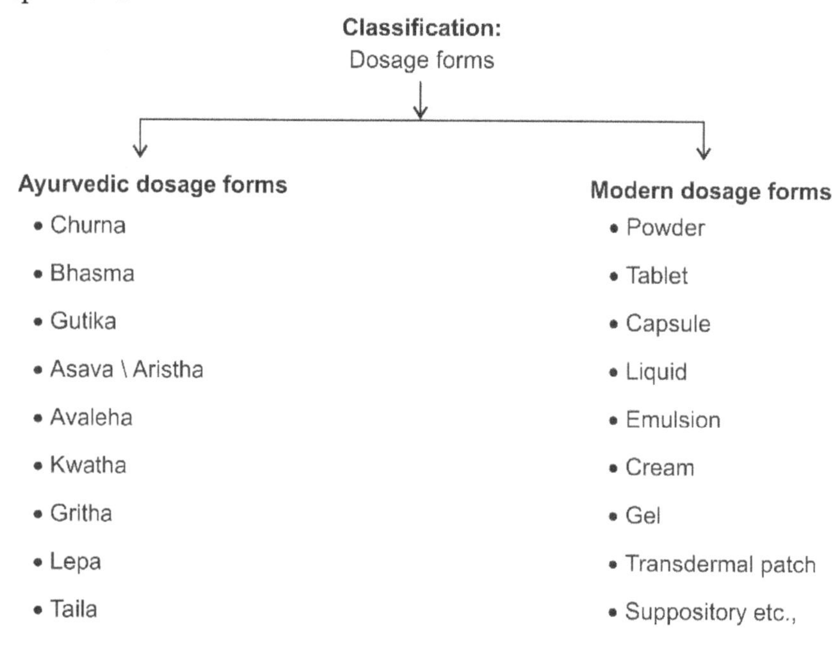

Method of preparation of 'Asava / Arishta'

Arishtas are made with decoctions of herbs in boiling water while asavas are prepared by directly by fresh herbal juices. This are unique liquid dosage forms that contain self-generated alcohol. Aristas and asavas are considered as a unique and valuable therapeutics in ayurveda due to their medical value, sweet taste and easy availability.

Preparation of Asava

- ➤ The drugs are coarsely powdered and kashay is prepared.
- ➤ Kashay is then prepared and kept in a fermentation pot.
- ➤ Sugar or jaggery are honey are dissolved and added to the solution after filtration.
- ➤ Finely powdered other drugs called as Prakshep dravya are added.
- ➤ Dhataki pushpa which is dried flower of a plant Woordfordia fructicoso is added at the end only.
- ➤ These flowers contain yeast which brings about fermentation of sugar present.
- ➤ The mouth of the pot, vessel or barrel is covered with earthen lid and the edges are sealed with clay-smeared cloth. Seven continuous layers of this cloth are used for covering.
- ➤ The pot is placed undisturbed in a heap of paddy to ensure fermentation.
- ➤ Temperature is maintained constant through out entire period. During this period bubbling sound can be heard from the pot due to releasing of gases.
- ➤ After some time remove the lid and the contents are examined whether the process is completed are not.
- ➤ The fluid is first decanted and then filtered after two or three days.
- ➤ If needed this process is repeated after boiling.

Preparation of Arishta

- ➤ Earthen pot used for fermentation should be old and properly cleaned. Fumigation with pipali churna should be done along with smearing with ghee.
- ➤ According to ayurvedic literature, self-generated alcohol acts as preservative so this preparation comes without expiry date.
- ➤ Jaggery or sugar is added to specific quantity of water, the mixture is boiled and cooled.
- ➤ After cooling the mixture is poured into fermentation pot.
- ➤ Finely powdered drugs are added to this liquid.

➢ Dhataki pushpa which is dried flower of a plant Woordfordia fructicoso is added at the end only, while the liquid is not hot.

➢ Further method of preparation of Arishta is same with preparation of Asava.

Gutika

Gutika is one of the simple ayurvedic medicines like pill or tablet. Gutika is palatable and easy to consume, store and preserve. There are many examples of gutika formulations.

Preparations

➢ First plant material is dried and made into fine powder.

➢ Other minerals, if mentioned in the formula are made into bhasma in fine powdered form.

➢ In some cases where mercury and sulphur are mentioned, Kajja (purified and consumable form of mercury and sulphur) is made first and other drugs are added to it, one by one.

➢ Mix the entire ingredients in mortar and pastel. Triturate herb, bhasma

➢ or other ingredients.

➢ Mix prescribed fluid to above mentioned ingredients to form soft paste.

➢ Add any other liquid mentioned, if any.

➢ When mass will convert into soft paste, additional aromatic and flavouring materials perfume can be added like Kasturi, Karpura.

➢ Triturate more to mix all the ingredients.

➢ Take non-sticky material while rolled to the fingers, make pills of required size by hand or pill making machine or automatic tablet punching machine.

➢ Dry the pill in shade or under sun according to requirement.

➢ Sugar or jaggery or Guggulu or Babool gum resin can be added as binder. In the case, binder should be added in liquid and then mixing is carried out.

e.g.: Chandraprabha vati, Eladi gutika, Dhanwanataram pills.

Lehya

Lehya is also known as Avaleh one of the several groups of Ayurvedic formulations. It is a semi-solid sugar-based preparation. It is prepared using sugar or jaggery or sugar candy and boiled with prescribed drug juice or decoction. Lehya is supposed to be taken with vehicle like water, goat milk, butter milk called as Anupan.

Preparation

> First sugar is dissolved into liquid medium, which can be water or juice. Liquids used in preparation of lehya may be decoction or expressed juice or hot infusion. Different types of sweetening agents can be used like sugar, jaggery, sugar candy, honey etc.

> The liquid containing sugar is heated and concentrated till 'paka' stage. At this stage concentrated semi-liquid will form into a thread when pressed between the thumb and index finger and released.

> Fine powder of drug is added into this mixture along with oil and ghee to get the semi-solid form. These are certain additives to increase potency of formulation called Prakshep dravya which can be herbal or metallic. Fat or oil added which works as Sneha dravya.

> Honey is added once the mixture is cooled. It is stirred further to get the appropriate semi-solid form.

> This is special formulation like medicated jam and should not be prepared overnight. Each avaleha need minimum of seven days to one month to mature.

> After preparation it should be kept in proper place for maturation.\

> There are two approaches for preparation:

- In first approach, juice or decoction is heated into a semi-solid paste and after those fine powders of the Prakshepa dravyas are added.

- In the second approach, jaggery or sugar is mixed with and heated till it becomes thick syrup followed by addition of prescribed drugs.

Precaution: Should be taken while addition of Prakshepa dravya. Prakshepa dravyas should be added at the end when preparation is hot. Sugandha dravya and Madhu should be added after cooling.

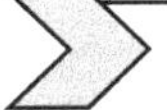

Bhasma

Bhasma is a calcinated preparation in which the gem or metal is converted into ash and complete burning or incineration. Gems or metals are first purified in order to remove impurities. Then they are triturated with herbal extracts. The resultant mass is calcinated and burned to obtain the ashes.

'Vibhuti' and 'Thiruneeru' are synonyms used for the bhasma. Bhasmikaran is process by which a substance which is otherwise bio-incompatible is most biocompatible by certain samskaras or processes.

Various steps involved in the preparation of bhasma are:

1. Shodhana – Purification
2. Marana – Size reduction or powdering

3. Chalan – stirring
4. Dhavna – washing
5. Galan – cleaning or filtering
6. Putan – heating
7. Mardan – triturating
8. Bhavana – coating with herbal extract
9. Amrutikaran – detoxification
10. Sandharan – preservation

Preparation

Sodhana can be done by washing of raw material, trituration, boiling with cow urine, milk, certain juice, reduction of toxic properties by triturating with certain juice or decoction, roasting, heating and quenching, melting of raw material and adding lime water or vegetable juice, distillation to remove impurities.

Marana it involves killing of metallic properties by several repeated steps.

Shodhana: The principle objective of shodhana is to remove unwanted part from the raw material and purification of metal. Metals obtained from ores may contain several impurities, sodhana is a process to remove impurities and making it suitable of next step.

Marana: Meaning of the word marana is killing. In this step, there is change in the chemical form or state of the metal. Because of this, metal lose its metallic characteristics and physical nature. Marana can be done with mercury, plants or sulphur. In shot after marana, metal can be converted into powder or other form suitable for administration. This step removes toxicity of metal used and make safe for consumption. Use of mercury is the most controversial topic according to the modern system of medicine, although it is considered as safe in ayurveda.

Chalan: Iron rod from specific plant is used for stirring hot metal. This process of stirring during heating the metal is called as chalan.

Dhavan: It involves washing with water to remove the excess amounts of agents used in shodhana or marana stage to remove water soluble constituents.

Galan: The product is then sifted either through a fine muslin cloth or through sieve, suitable mesh so as to separate residual material larger in size.

Puttan: This is key step in preparation of bhasma. The term puttan means heating in special earthen vessel or pot. Generally, shallowness of vessel is useful in heating of the material faster and uniformly. After keeping the material on the material on the shallow surface the part is used as a lid, by placing it in an invented position. Puttan can be of different types depending on nature of process like chandraputa, dhanyarashiputta, suryaputta, bhugarbhaputta, agniputta.

Churna: It is defined as a fine powder of one or more drugs. Churna formulation is similar to powder formulation in Allopathic system of medicine. Churna should be given with some other vehicle like honey, milk or sugar, this make administration of churna easy and increased palatability also enchances therapeutic effect.

Preparation

- ❖ Plant material is collected and cleaned.
- ❖ Plant material is dried in shade or sun according to specific requirements.
- ❖ Dried material is pulverized and then sieved through mesh 60 or 80.
- ❖ Finally, it is stored in well closed container on proper place.

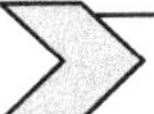 **Taila**

These are preparations consisting of lipophilic liquid in the form of medicated oil. They are meant for external use.

Preparation:

Taila is prepared by dissolving or extracting the medicated substances with an oil like mustard oil.

CHAPTER 8

Role of Medicinal and Aromatic Plants in National Economy and their Export Potential

Since ancient times, mankind has relied mostly on the plant kingdom to suit all of its medicinal needs: for treating illnesses, seeking eternal health, longevity, and seeking relief from pain and discomfort, as well as for aroma, favours and delicacies. It had motivated early man to investigate his immediate natural surroundings and experiment with a wide range of plant, animal, and mineral items, as well as develop a variety of therapeutic treatments.

Because medicines are vital to sustaining a healthy community that drives and sustains the economy, medicinal plants remain critical and strategic to the economies of low-income countries. To achieve any level of self-reliance in terms of availability of effective and safe medications for the management of recurrent illness conditions in such low-income nations, policy directional change is required. Because of the significance of self in the present and possibly future economically and politically intrigues involving wealthy countries in the medicines sector, this transformation must be prioritised.

Despite improvements in modern Western medicine, medicinal plants continue to play an essential role in both preventive and curative therapies in Asia's emerging and developing countries. They also provide money to residents in several Asian countries, who make a living by selling forest-collected items or cultivating crops on their farms.

As a result, medicinal plants are a valuable national resource. Plants have been used in organised health care systems in India and China for over 5,000 years. Herbal medicines grew in popularity in Europe throughout the Graeco-Roman period and were popular until the 1960s.

India, China, Greece, the Arab world, and other ancient civilizations established their own systems of medicine, but they were all primarily plant-based. However, ayurveda outperformed organised systems of medicine in terms of theoretical underpinning and in-depth understanding of medical practise. It is possibly the oldest (6,000 B.C.) of the structured traditional medical systems. People from all around the world use it.

According to the World Health Organization (WHO), traditional medicines, predominantly plant pharmaceuticals, are used by 80 percent of the population in underdeveloped nations for basic health care. Even today's pharmacopoeia comprises at least 25% of medications originated from plants, as well as several semisynthetic drugs based on prototype compounds extracted from plants. Medicinal plants are an important part of all indigenous and alternative medicine systems. They are used in ayurveda, homoeopathy, naturopathy, Oriental, and Native American Indian medicine, for example.

Herbal pharmaceuticals are becoming more popular around the world as people recognise the benefits of natural plant-based remedies, which are nontoxic, have no side effects, are readily available at low prices, and are sometimes the sole source of health care for the poor.

Approximately 90% of the medicinal plants utilised in the industry are taken from the wild. Only about 20 plant species are commercially grown, despite the fact that industries use over 800 kinds. Because of unsustainable use of these medicinal plants results in a serious threat to the genetic stock and diversity of medicinal plant resources, as well as the country's economy, if biodiversity is not managed sustainably.

The WHO launched a campaign to raise awareness about the importance and usefulness of traditional and indigenous herbal medicine. Its efforts in the 1970s resulted in an appeal to all member countries to do everything possible to preserve their national heritage in the form of ethnomedicine and ethnopharmacology, as well as to reinstate the use of known and tested medicinal plants and derivatives in primary health care in rural areas as alternatives to modern medicines when modern medicines are unavailable.

According to a WHO survey from 2003, 30 percent of medications supplied worldwide comprised substances derived from plant materials, with global herbal product sales estimated to be worth 600 million dollars in 2002. Plant-based medications are used by 80 percent of the populace in underdeveloped countries for their healthcare requirements. As a result, the commercial aspect of medicinal plant use is likely to provide an incentive and a major development strategy to best protect the interests of low-income countries. Interest in medicinal herbs as a re-emerging medical aid has been spurred by the increasing prices of drugs drugs in the maintenance of general health and well-being, as well as the "bio-prospecting" of novel plant-derived pharmaceuticals, as observed by the Bank Group and later Hoareau and DaSilva.

Plant-derived prescription medications have been tipped as the next large business development in biotechnology because of the advantages they offer in terms of scale production and economy, product safety, easiness of storage and distribution, and they also offer the most promising future to supply reduced prescription medications to the developing world.

Plants have long been employed in India for medical and animal health care, as well as in the textile and food industries. Ninety percent of indigenous people's local food resources were unknown to nutrient literature, trade, cosmetics, and perfumes; however, India holds a unique position in the field of herbal medicine, as one of the few countries capable of cultivating almost all of the important species used in both modern and traditional medicine. This is due to India's large size and diversity in climate, soil, altitude/latitude, and flora.

The herbal drug market as a whole is rising at a pace of 20% to 30% per year, with various companies reporting different growth rates. The government's strategy of supporting makers of solely herbal goods can also be credited with the market's strong development rate. This is compounded by the lack of any pricing guidelines. Pricing guidelines for ethical medications, unlike the 'Drug Price Control Order (DPCO),' have resulted in this market being seen as a highly attractive option source of revenue. The herbal market has benefited from the new patents policy under the 'GATT,' which went into force in 2005.

Plants are the primary source of alternative medicines in underdeveloped countries. According to the World Health Organization, up to 80% of the world's people rely on the traditional remedies for their primary care, the majority of which employ plant-based therapies. Traditional medicine is becoming more popular in developing countries as the population grows. The government seeks to support indigenous medicine rather than relying on imported pharmaceuticals, and there are significant attempts to revitalise traditional cultures; simple access and cost efficiency have an impact on the national economy.

In 1995, the yearly turnover of the herbal sector in India was expected to be over US\$ 250 million. According to a Chemexcil report, the value of Ayurveda medicine exported in 1999–2000 was roughly US\$ 41.6 million, with the top OTC products contributing approximately US\$ 30.5 million.

The need for therapeutic plants in India, which includes 162 species, is predicted to rise by 15 to 16 percent between 2002 and 2005 to meet both export and domestic markets. According to evidence, India's total national potential for crude pharmaceuticals and oil extracts is worth Rs 3 billion, with the need for over-the-counter products accounting for half of that. Cosmetics, ethical and classical formulation, and ethical and classic formulations each account for Rs 1.2 billion, whilst traditional Vaidya medicines and herbal remedial formulations account for Rs 400 million and Rs 200 million, respectively. As a result, medicinal plant production and management could become financially and economically lucrative for small-scale growers.

The economic importance of therapeutic plants is increasing. In order to strengthen their economic and health-care delivery systems, developing countries must harness. The "pharmerging" countries appear to be aware of the financial dynamics and are rising to the occasion. In particular, developing nations in the African region must make greater efforts to address these health and financial challenges, particularly in light of the resurgence and emergence of resistant pathogenic microorganisms and cancers, which have become a serious threat to our unified survival.

CHAPTER 9

Nutraceuticals

Hippocrates accurately highlighted "Let food be your medicine and medicine be your diet" almost 2000 years ago. Due to the realisation that "nutraceuticals" have a significant role in health enhancement, there is currently a rise in global 14 interest. Dr. Stephen DeFelice, the chairman of the Foundation for Innovation in Medicine, combined the words "nutrition" and "pharmaceutical" to create the phrase

A dietary product that is marketed with the intention of treating or preventing disease is referred to as a nutraceutical. This phrase lacks any regulatory definition. Therefore, a "nutraceutical" would be any substance that might be categorised as food or a component of food that has medical or health advantages, including the prevention of illness.

"Nutraceuticals and functional foods have received considerable interest because of their presumed safety and potential nutritional and therapeutic effects".

Food is referred to as "functional food" when it is prepared or cooked with "scientific intelligence," whether or not the user is aware of how or why the food is being used. As a result, functional food gives the body the essential amount of vitamins, lipids, proteins, and carbohydrates for a healthy existence. A "nutraceutical" is a functional food that assists mostly in prevention or treatment of disease more that 15 deficient conditions like anaemia.

Recent research has indicated that these chemicals may be effective in treating a variety of pathological consequences, including cancer, diabetes, atherosclerosis, cardiovascular diseases (CVDs), and neurological disorders. These circumstances bring about a variety of modifications, including redox state changes. The majority of dietary supplements have antioxidant activity that can help to prevent this condition. As a result, they are regarded as beneficial sources for promoting health, particularly in terms of preventing fatal conditions like diabetes, infections, renal, and digestive illnesses.

In order to facilitate comprehension and use, nutraceuticals can be arranged in a variety of ways, such as for dietary recommendations, clinical trial design, or academic training. Nutraceuticals can be categorised in a variety of ways, such as according to their dietary origins, mode of action, chemical makeup, etc. All-natural food sources that are employed as nutraceuticals include the following:

- Dietary fibres
- Pre-biotics
- Pro-biotics
- Polyunsaturated fatty acids
- Anti-oxidants
- Polyphenols
- Spices

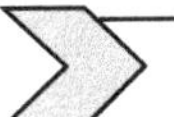 **Dietary Fibres**

Dietary fibre is any meal or, more specifically, any plant material, that is not hydrolyzed by digestive tract enzymes but rather is digested by gut bacteria. Non-starch polysaccharide (NSP) such cellulose, hemicellulose, gums, and pectin, as well as lignin, resistant dextrin, and resistant starches, make up the majority of dietary fibres. Fruits, oats, barley, and beans are foods high in soluble fibre. In terms of chemistry, dietary fibre refers to carbohydrate polymers with such a degree of polymerization of at least 3 that neither are digested nor absorbed from the gastrointestinal.

Examples: Apples, bananas, carrots, cabbage, white bread, brown bread etc.,

Therapeutic applications

- ➤ Soluble fibre has been demonstrated to improve glucose tolerance, promote insulin receptor binding, and reduce serum LDL cholesterol in a selective manner.
- ➤ Dietary fibre promotes faecal bulking in the colon because it increases water retention, transit duration, and faecal bacterial mass due to the fermentation of soluble fibre.
- ➤ People who consume large levels of dietary fibre had lower risks of stroke, hypertension, diabetes, obesity, and several gastrointestinal problems than people who consume little or no fibre.
- ➤ An increase in the consumption of high-fibre foods helps with weight loss, decreases blood pressure, and improves blood glucose management in diabetics.

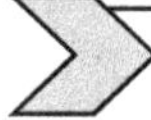

Probiotics

Probiotics are live microbial feed supplements that, when given to animals in sufficient doses, improve the balance of the bacteria in their intestines. The following types of bacteria are typically found in probiotics: lactobacilli, gram-positive cocci, and bifidobacteria.

Applications

> ➤ Probiotics are typically used to treat gastrointestinal (GI) issues include lactose intolerance, severe diarrhoea, and GI side effects from antibiotics.

> ➤ Probiotic agents are non-pathogenic, non-toxic, resistant to gastric acid, and able to cling to gut epithelial tissues, where they produce antibacterial compounds.

> ➤ Administration of probiotics lowers the risk of systemic illnesses like allergies, asthma, cancer, and a number of other ear and urinary tract infections.

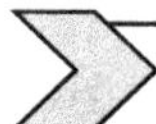

Prebiotics

Prebiotics are compounds in food that induce the growth or activity of beneficial microorganisms such as bacteria and fungi.There is a strong correlation between the immune system and the health of gastrointestinal tract, as about 70%-80% of all immune cells are present in the gut. When prebiotics are consumed at an early stage, they create conditions in the gut that are optimum to train the immune system.

Applications

> ➤ The prebiotic consumption generally promotes the Lactobacillus and Bifidobacterial growth in the gut, thus helping in metabolism.

> ➤ Improved lactose tolerance, anticancer capabilities, toxin neutralisation, stimulation of the gut immune system, reduction of constipation, blood lipids, and blood cholesterol levels are only a few of the health advantages of prebiotics.

> ➤ Breast milk contain large amount of prebiotics which helps child to grow healthy and reduce bad bacteria count.

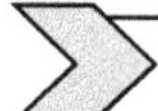

Anti-oxidants and Carotenoids

Vitamins like vitamin C, E, and carotenoids are referred to as antioxidant vitamins combined. These vitamins, which are plentiful in many fruits and vegetables, work through free-radical scavenging systems to protect us from harm. Citrus fruits, grains, nuts, oils, tomatoes, oranges, and more examples.

Applications

> ➢ Prevents the damage caused by free radicals to the body's cells, thereby promoting longevity and warding off disease.

> ➢ Scavenging free radicals and chelating metal ions.

Health Advantages

- Because nutraceuticals are natural dietary supplements, they have less negative effects.

- The use of nutraceuticals improves human health and improves medical conditions.

- It is widely available and reasonably priced, i.e. cost-effective.

- Nutraceuticals aid in the detoxification of the body.

- It aids in the prevention of vitamin and mineral deficits.

- It aids in the restoration of proper digestion and eating habits.

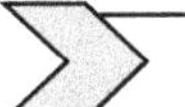 **Spirulina**

Biological source

It is obtained from the plant *Spindina platensis* belonging to the family Oscillatoriaceae.

Chemical constituents

Gamma linoleic acid, oleic acid, glycol-proteins, sulpholipids.

Use as a nutraceutical product

It is a dietary supplement. Antioxidant that helps to prevent diseases brought on by free radicals. Thyroid gland stimulant, Immune system and prostaglandin levels stimulation, Probiotics are beneficial to the body's resistance, Atherosclerosis prevention, platelet aggregation prevention, blood vessel dilation prevention, xerophthalmia, cataract prevention, and night blindness prevention, Treatment of cancer, pancreatitis, cirrhosis, and hepatitis with a therapeutic supplement. Diabetes management, Adults, athletes, growing and malnourished youngsters should take a dietary supplement.

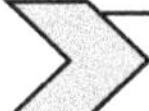 **Soya**

Biological source: It is obtained from Glycine max belonging to the family

Leguminosea.

Chemical constituents

Daidzein, genistein

Use as a nutraceutical product

Soybean is utilised as a raw material for oil milling, and soy waste is used as animal feed. Soybeans are high in nutritional value. Soy sauce, miso, natto, yoghurts, kinako, protein crisp, sweets, baby food, and soy milk are all examples of fermented and non fermented soy products. For various illnesses, such as lactose intolerance and severe gastroenteritis in babies, soybean base products are used as a primary protein source. Soybean protein has an adequate number of essential amino acids such as histidine, isoleucine, leucine, lysine, phenylalanine, tyrosine, threonine, tryptophan, and valine, all of which are recommended for daily consumption as part of a balanced diet. It is said to provide various health benefits, including decreasing plasma cholesterol, preventing cancer, increasing bone mineral density, and providing energy.

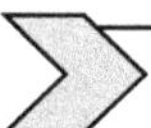# Garlic

Biological source: It is obtained from the bulbs of Allium sativum belonging to the family Liliaceae.

Chemical constituents: Allicin, allin and Ajoene.

Uses: To treat hyperlipidaemia, it have antihypertensive, hypoglycemic, anti-spasmodic activity, prevent colon and lung cancer. It's a Most Potent Superfood as the research states that 63% lower risk of catching the virus due to 'allin', a well-known immunity booster. It aids in weight loss. It is used as a Blood Pressure Lowering Agent, As a Cure to Alzheimer's and Dementia due to presence of phenolic compounds. Increases Athletic Performance as it provides an instant surge of energy and vigour. Garlic can increase a person's life span significantly.

CHAPTER 10

Herbal Formulations

Herbal remedies have been employed in traditional medicinal practices. While herbal medicine practitioners are generally comfortable with their use and are generally convinced by the effects they see with clients, the scientific relevance of herbal remedies in research and innovation is still being debated. This is due in part to a lack of quality assurance, identification, and standardization of compounds and drug formulations, and the difficulties of applying the same methodology to different pharmaceutical goods. Herbal medicine's development within the context of evidence-based therapy is relatively new. The research community faces a complex set of obstacles when it comes to applying the methodology of Western-based pharmaceutical sciences to natural remedies.

Herbal medicine research must, however, be designed and conducted in a scientific and ethical manner, while also taking into consideration the medical beliefs and practices that accompany the use of traditional herbal therapy.

Herbal formulations are now widely used in the pharma health care system for treat a variety of ailments. Phytotherapy has a lengthy history dating back thousands of years. The advent of herbs and plants in the popular dietary supplement and nutraceuticals is another factor driving market share and popularity. The use of phytotherapeutics has increased considerably among patients and professionals, as indicated by an increasing market for herbal treatments. Because of their extensive biological activity, higher safety margins, and lower costs, herbal drugs are in considerable demand for primary health care both in developed and developing countries. Since all constituents are active, the therapeutic impact of herbal drugs is based on the total function of a variety of active components.

Challenges facing with Herbal formulations:

- The impartial assessment of contradicting toxicological, epidemiological, and other data, as well as the authentication of herbal materials employed, is a major difficulty.

- Risk management within risk ranges

- Uncertainty communication

- Documentation on pharmacology, toxicology, and clinical care
- Pharmacovigilance
- Herbal Formulation Challenges
- Understanding why hazardous chemicals work and analysing "drug" interactions are important.
- Clinical trial constraints and the number of persons available
- Standardization
- Assessment of safety and efficacy.

Herbs are available in a wide range of contemporary pharmaceutical formulations, include tablets, capsule, topical ointments, gels, and ointments, and some unusual drug delivery formats like sustained release and microcapsules dosage forms.

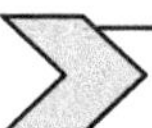 **Dosage Forms**

Infusion:

- The dilute solutions of the readily soluble constituents of crude drugs are called infusions.

The infusion is prepared by:

- 2-3gm of dried or fresh herb is placed in the strainer of the cup tisane.
- Freshly boiled water is taken in the cup.
- Close the lip of the cup and infuse for 5-10minutes prior removing the strainer.
- Finally add the sweetner, if desired.

  For Ex:

  Cinnamon infusion for antitussive property,

  Mint infusion and Vitamin C for vitamins.

Decoctions

The plant constituents are made solubilized in water by boiling the desired herb in vehicle like water for a definite time, cooled and filtered is known as decoction.

The decoction is prepared by

- Fresh or dried form of drug in a saucepan.
- Fill the saucepan with cold water and subject for boiling.
- Boil for 20-30minutes, till the reduction of 500ml.
- Strain the liquid and store in a cool place.

For Ex:

Calumba decoction, Corydalis decoction, Astragalus decoction and Ginger decoction.

Tinctures

These are the solutions containing medicinal substances in conc or dil. Alcohol.

The tinctures are prepared by

Fresh or dried drug is taken in 35-40% of acohol in jar. Shake it well.

Store in a cool dark place for 10-14 days.

Pass through nylon mesh.

Transfer the filterated tincture to dark glass bottle.

For Ex:

Strophanthus tincture and pepper tincture.

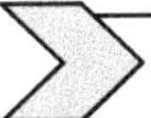 **Capsules**

Powders are prepared for the preparation of Capsules.

Capsules are prepared by

Select the herbs desired for the formulating the herbal capsule.

Dry the herbs and make powder.

Fill the powder in halves of the capsule and fix the both halves of the capsule.

For Ex:

Buchu capsule for the treatment of cystitis and myrrh capsule for bronchial catarrh.

Medicated wines:

The wines are also called as tonic wines.

They are agreeable which increases vitality and improve digestion.

Medicated wines are prepared by

Take fresh or dried drug in cleaned jar. Pour the desired amount of wine.

All the wine to get mature for the period of 2 weeks.

Regularly top up the mixture with wine.

For Ex:

Madeira red wine for digestive problems and rosemary leaves wine for nervous problems.

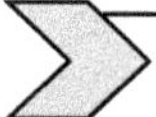

Syrups

A syrup is prepared by equal proportions of a herbal infusion or decoction by adding up honey or unrefined sugar.

Syrup is prepared by

- Take an infusion or decoction in a pan.
- Add a sufficient quantity f honey or sugar.
- Heat for specific period of time with constant stirring till the desired consistency is acheived.
- Remove from heat and cool.
- Pour the cooled syrup in the container.

  For Ex:

  Raspberry syrup and Cherry Syrup

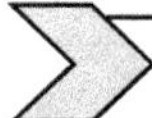

Tablets

Tablets are solid dosage forms of powdered herbs or herbal extracts or their constituents prepared by compression.

It is prepared by

- Herbal drugs are selected, dried, fine powdered and pass through sieve no. 100.
- All the medicaments and excipients are mixed uniformly.
- The mixed ingredients are made into granulation by wet or dry granulation.
- The compressed granules are made into tablets.
- The tablets are coated and subjected for evaluated.

  For Ex:

  Tablet for acute fever consists of Tabasheer, quinine bark, tinospora and gum acacia.

  Table for Jaundice consists of Aloe, Cocklebur, myrobalan and wild celery.

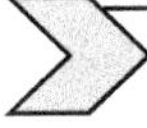 **Ointments**

These are the semi-solid dosage forms meant for external application to the skin or mucous membrane.

The prepared ointment should be stable, smooth, free from grittiness, melt or soften at body temperature.

It is prepared by:

Melt the wax by placing it in a pan of boiling water.

Add the fine powder of herb and heat for 15 min. for boiling.

Filter and squeeze and transfer the molten ointment into jar.

For Ex:

Juniper berry ointment and Calcium carbonate ointment.

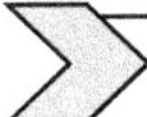 **Creams**

They are viscous semi-solid ointment like preparations.

It can be prepared by

Wax is melted in a pan by boiling water.

Strain the mixture and transfer it into a dark glass jar. Tighten the lid and store in a refrigerator.

The bioavailability of most herbal preparations is low. Novel delivery systems such as phytosomes, liposomes, marinosomes, niosomes, and photosomes, among others, can be used to circumvent this constraint. These technologies can increase the efficacy of distribution as well as the ability to traverse lipid-rich biomembranes, overcoming the limits of standard drug delivery systems.

Some of the conventional Herbal Dosage forms are:

(a) Phytosome

In comparison to traditional herbal extracts, phytosomes are enhanced types of herbal supplements that are more absorbed, utilised, and can offer superior effects. When used to herbal medications and phytoconstituents, modern drug delivery technologies will offer up new pathways for maximising the medicinal potential of polar plant compounds.

(b) Niosome

The membranous structure of the new drug delivery system, in which the herbal medication is enclosed in a vesicle, is tiny. Niosome surfactants are nonimmunogenic, biodegradable, and biocompatible. However, medication transport via the transdermal route appears to suggest that more fluid membranes are more efficient. Vesicle length has not been thoroughly described, and investigations are being conducted to rigorously determine the standards and requirements for specific pharmacodynamic purposes.

(c) Liposomes

Liposomes are colloidal vesicles that are spherical in shape and self-closed. They have a bilayer of phospholipids in their interior that adsorbs part of the solvents wherein they freely float. In the event of a single bilayer encasing the aqueous core, tiny or big unilamellar vesicles are defined, whereas in the case of several concentric bilayers, only huge multilamellar vesicles are defined.

(d) Photosomes

Photosomes are made up of liposomes that include photolyases (a bacterial enzyme that can repair UVB-induced cyclobutane pyrimidine dimers (CPD) in eukaryotes). Photolyases are enzyme that can bind to a lesion and use light energy to reverse the damage through photo reactivation. Photolyases are 50–60 kDa monomeric flavoproteins with two chromophores as co - factors. These photo reactivating enzymes utilise the energy of near UV/visible light (300–500 nm) to rebuild CPD or 6-4 photoproducts directly and effectively.

Herbal drugs have a lot of therapeutic promise, and there should be further research into value-added drug delivery techniques. The two most critical determinants for poor performance, limited bioavailability, and absorption are the mobility of lipids as well as the structure of their molecules. When delivered utilising a novel drug delivery vehicle, standardised phytoconstituents or polar phytoconstituents including flavonoid, terpenoids, tannins, and xanthones get a significantly better absorption profile, allowing them to pass through the biological barrier and boost bioavailability. Site-specific controlled release can also be achieved using new formulations.

CHAPTER 11

Herbal Cosmetics

The word "cosmetic" comes from the Greek word "kosm tikos," which means "power to arrange, skill to decorate." As cosmetics have evolved, they have formed a continuous narrative throughout man's history. In prehistoric times (3000BC), man employed colours to attract the animals he wanted to hunt, as well as to withstand enemy attacks by color his skin and adorning his physique for protection and to induce fear in an opponent (whether man or animal). Cosmetics have been linked to hunting, fighting, religion, and superstition in the past, and are now linked to medicine.

The information was eventually separated from medicine and transferred to pharmacy. The ancient man had a magical suggestion for dazzling others with their beauty; there have been no beauty creams or cosmetic surgery to change one's look at the time. The skin and hair beauty is dependent on health and lifestyle. Exposure towards heat results in dryness of skin, brings up wrinkles, pigmentation and sunburns on skin.   Apart from these cracks, wounds and infections are very common side effects during winter times.

Skin illnesses due to exposure to bacteria, chemical agents, biological toxins in the environment results in aging in people. The understanding of nature accumulated in the ayurveda was the only thing they would have to rely on. Many herbs and floras were used in ayurvedic cosmetics for attractiveness and prevention from external influences. The botanicals' natural content has no negative impact on the body body; rather, it enriches it with nutrition and other beneficial minerals.

Cosmetics are defined as articles meant to be rubbed, poured, sprinkled, sprayed on, introduced into, and otherwise administered to the human body or any portion thereof for washing, rejuvenating, enhancing attractiveness, or altering the appearance, according the Drugs and Cosmetics Act. The cosmetic is not covered by a drug licence preview. Herbal cosmetics are products that contain phytochemicals extracted from a number of plant sources affects skin functions and enriches nutrient value to bring out skin and hair healthy. The usage of plant originated products in cosmetics are high due to their aromatic value.

Recently, a vast variety of cosmetics and toiletry formulations based on Indian herbs have been produced. Aside from the traditional uses, some recent studies have demonstrated the efficacy of Indian botanicals in Consumer Care products. Herbal Cosmetics, sometimes known as Products, are developed with a variety of legal cosmetic components to form the base, and one or more herbal substances are employed and provide stated cosmetic benefits solely.

Herbal treatments are becoming increasingly popular due to their absence of adverse effects. The nicest part about beauty products is that they are produced entirely of herbs and shrubs. The natural composition of the herbs has no adverse effects on human body; rather, it enriches it with nutrients as well as other beneficial minerals. Cosmetic products are defined as any substance used for various external parts of body according to European Directives 93/35/EEC (European Commission).

Plants, on the other hand, now have a wide and complex arsenal of active ingredients (photochemicals) capable of not only calming and smoothing the skin, but also actively restoring, healing, and protecting it.

Herbal Cosmetic	Source	Chemical constituents	Commercial Preparations	Therapeutic Uses & Cosmetic Uses
Aloe vera	Aloe is the dried juice obtained from the leaves of various species of Aloe like *Aloe perryi, Aloe vera,* and *Aloe barbadensis* belonging to the family Liliaceae.	Aloin is the chief constituent of aloes it is the mixture of 3 isomers namely barbaloin, iso-barbaloin, β-barbaloin, glycosides, anthracene. Aloin A (Barbaloin) Aloin B (Isobarbaloin)	Gels, soaps, ointments, capsules, aloe vera juice, sun creams, shampoos, etc.	• Used as laxative and purgative. • Used to treat burns, acne, pimples and psoriasis. • Used in cosmetics. • Used in hair fall. • Treat irregular menstrual cycles. • Treatment of obesity.

Table *Contd...*

Herbal Cosmetic	Source	Chemical constituents	Commercial Preparations	Therapeutic Uses & Cosmetic Uses
Almond Oil	Almond oil is a fixed oil obtained by expression from the seeds of *Prunus amygdalus* belonging to the family Rosacea.	Oleic acid, Palmitic acid, Palmitoleic acid, Benzaldehyde, Stigmasterol, Isofucosterol, Campesterol and Avenasterol	Hair oil, Skin oil and Sweet almond oil	• Memory enhancement • Reduce cholesterol • It acts as immune modulator • Inhalation of almond oil relaxes nerves and smoothen anxiety. • It treats black heads and dark circles. • Used to relieve tooth pain • Flavouring agent
Olive Oil	It is obtained from the fruit of the *Olea europea* belonging to the family Oleaceae.	It contains glycerides of oleic acid, palmitic, linoleic, stearic and myristic acids.	Eye Cream, Body Scrub, Makeup Remover, Hair Serum, Overnight Lip Mask and Hair Conditioner.	• It is used as emollient. • It is used in the manufacturing of creams, lotions, bath oils. • Used to treat heart diseases, high blood pressure.
Rosemary Oil	Oil of Rosemary is distilled from the flowering tops of leafy twigs of *Rosmarinus officinalis* belonging to family Lamiaceae.	1,8-cineole, borneol, camphor, bornyl acetate, and monoterpene hydrocarbons are the principal constituents. The leaves contains triterpene alcohols α- and β-amyrins, rosmarinic acid, caffeic acid, chlorogenic acid. It also contains glycosides namely luteolin and diosmetin, carnosolic acid, carnosol, rosmanol, etc.,	Anti-Dandruff Hair Oil, Anti-Dandruff Shampoo and Protein Shampoo for oily/greasy hair. Erina Plus (Himalaya Drug Company).	• It is used in aromatherapy • During gastrointestinal disturbances, Enhances urinary and digestive elimination. • Clears nasal passages, colds. • Used in mouthwashes and for rheumatic ailments. • It is used in food technology as it posses antioxidant activity..

Table *Contd...*

Herbal Cosmetic	Source	Chemical constituents	Commercial Preparations	Therapeutic Uses & Cosmetic Uses
		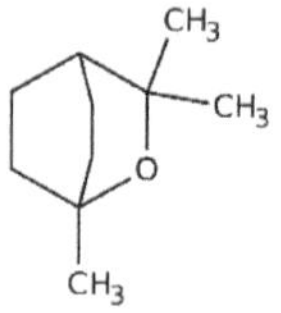 **1,8- Cineole** 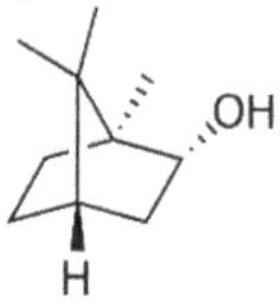 **Borneol**		
Sandalwood Oil	It is obtained from the steam of *Santalum album* (Indian sandalwood) and *Santalum spicatum* (Australian sandalwood) belonging to the family Santalaceae.	Medicinal constituent of Sandal-wood is santalol. 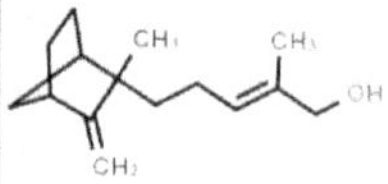 **Santalol** It consists of two isomers - α-santalol and β-santalol.	Evecare, Lukol, Antiwrinkle cream by Himalaya Drug Company and Brahma rasayan (Dabur).	• It is extensively used in perfumery as they were used in toiletry products. • It is chemo-protective in nature.

CHAPTER 12

Preliminary Phytochemical Screening

The plant is a biosynthetic laboratory synthesizes chemical compounds like carbohydrates, proteins and lipids that are utilized by man and also a multitude of compounds like glycosides, alkaloids, volatile oils, tannins etc., that exert a physiological and therapeutic effect. The compounds that are responsible for medicinal property of the drug are usually secondary metabolites. The plant material of a crude drug is subjected to preliminary phytochemical screening for the detection of various plant constituents.

Chemical tests were carried out on the aqueous extract and on the powdered specimens using standard procedures to identify the constituents

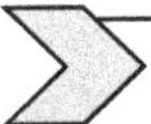 ## Tests for Primary Metabolites of Plants

Chemical tests for Carbohydrates

Test	Observation	Inference
1. **Molisch test:** To the sample solution add Molisch reagent and conc. H_2SO_4 from the sides of the test tube	A purple coloured ring is formed at the junction of two layers	Presence of reducing sugars.
2. **Fehling's test:** To the test solution add Fehling's A and B solution about 1ml and boil on water bath.	Brick red precipitate is formed	Presence of reducing sugars.
3. **Benedict's test:** To the test solution add 2ml Benedict's reagent and boil on water bath for 5 minutes	Red coloured precipitate is formed	Presence of reducing sugars.
4. **Barfoed's test:** To the test solution add 2ml of Barfoed's reagent and boil.	Brick red precipitate is formed at the bottom.	Presence of monosaccharide.
5. **Seliwanoff's test:** To the test solution add seliwan off's reagent and boil	A dark pink colour is produced	Presence of pentose.
6. A solution of the sample is heated with equal volume of hydrochloric acid containing a little phloroglucinol	A red colour is produced	Presence of pentose.

Test for non-reducing sugars

1. Test solution does not give response to Fehling's and Benedict's tests.
2. Hydrolyse test solution then Fehling's and Benedict's tests give positive response.

Test for non-reducing polysaccharides (starch):

Iodine test: Mix 3ml test solution and few drops of dilute iodine solution. Blue colour appears which disappears on boiling and reappears on cooling.

Tannic acid test for starch: With 20% tannic acid, test solution gives precipitate.

Test for gums

Hydrolyse test solution using dilute HCl. Perform Fehling's or Benedict's test. Red colour is developed.

Test for mucilage

1. Powdered drug material shows red colour with ruthenium red.
2. Powdered drug swells in water or aqueous KOH.

Test for Proteins

1. **Biuret test (General test):** Mix 2 ml of test solution with 4 % w/v NaOH and add 1 % w/v $CuSO_4$ solution drop by drop. Purplish violet or pinkish violet colour appears.
2. **Ferric chloride test:** To 2 ml of protein solution, add ferric chloride solution drop by drop. A white precipitate or turbidity developed.
3. **Millon's test:** To 2 ml of sample solution add equal volume of millon's reagent (10 % mercuric sulphate in 10 % H_2SO_4) and boil the contents, cool it and finally add few drops of 1 % w/v sodium nitrite and warm it again. Deep red colour solution formed indicates the presence of tyrosine.
4. **Xanthoproteic test (proteins containing tyrosine and tryptophan):** Mix 3 ml of sample solution with 1 ml of concentrated HNO_3, Boil the contents and cool. Precipitate turns to yellow. Add NaOH till it become alkaline, precipitate turns to orange. Indicates the presence of aromatic amino acids.
5. **Test for protein containing sulphur:** Mix 5 ml sample solution with 2 ml of 40 % NaOH. Boil the contents and add two drops of 10 % lead acetate solution. Black or brownish precipitate is formed due to lead sulphide (PbS)
6. **Precipitation test:** The test solution gives white colloidal precipitate with following reagents
   (i) Absolute alcohol.

(ii) 5 % $HgCl_2$ solution.

(iii) 5 % $CuSO_4$ solution.

(iv) 5 % lead acetate.

(v) 5 % ammonium sulphate.

7. **Ninhydrin test (general test for amino acids):** To 2 ml of protein solution add 1 ml of 0.2 % Ninhydrin solution and boil the contents slightly for 5 minutes in a boiling water bath. Purple or violet colour is observed.

Test for fixed oils and fats

1. Small quantity of the extract was pressed between two filter papers; permanent oil stain on the paper indicates the presence of fixed oil.

2. **Saponification test**: Few drops of 0.5 N alcoholic potassium hydroxide is added to small quantity of extract along with a drop of phenolphthalein. The mixture was heated on water bath for 1-2 hours. Formation of soap or partial neutralization of alkali indicates the presence of fixed oil and fats.

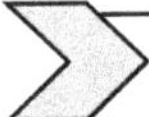 **Tests for Secondary Metabolites of Plants**

Test for Alkaloids

- Evaporate the aqueous, alcoholic or chloroform extracts separately, to the residue add dil. HCl. Shake well and filter with filtrate and perform following tests.

  1. Alcoholic extract + **Dragendroff's reagent** (solution of potassium bismuth iodide) → reddish brown precipitate.

  2. Alcoholic extract + **Wagner's reagent** (solution of iodine in potassium iodide) → reddish brown precipitate.

  3. Alcoholic extract + **Mayer's reagent** (potassium mercuric iodide) → cream coloured precipitate.

  4. Alcoholic extract + **Hager's reagent** (saturated solution of picric acid) → yellow coloured precipitate.

- These reagents also give precipitate with proteins.

- Caffeine and other purine derivatives do not respond to above tests and can be detected by Murexide test.

- Indole alkaloids (ex Ergot) give bluish violet or red colour with H_2SO_4 and p-dimethyl aminobenzaldehyde (van-urk's reagent).

  Tropane alkaloids → Vitali - Morin test.

  Colchicine + Mineral acids → yellow colour.

Triterpenoids

1. **Libermann's test:** Mix 3 ml plant extract solution with 2 ml acetic anhydride, heated and cooled down. 2 drops of concentrated H_2SO_4 is added. Blue colour indicates the presence of triterpenes.

2. **Libermann & Burchard's test:** 2 ml of plant extract is mixed with chloroform; add 1-2 ml of acetic anhydride and 2 drops of concentrated H_2SO_4 from the sides of the test tube. First red, then blue and finally green colour appears. This is test for steroids.

3. **Salkowski test:** To the chloroform extract, few ml of concentrated H_2SO_4 is added. Appearance of red colour at the interface indicates the presence of triterpenes.

Test for Phenolics/ tannins

1. Extract + $FeCl_3$ → intense blackish blue colour formation.

2. Extract +10 % solution of lead acetate + water → white coloured precipitate.

3. **Gelatin test:** solutions of tannins (about 0.5 to 1.0 %) precipitate a 1 % solution of gelatin containing 10 % NaCl.

Test for Glycosides

Drug powder is hydrolyzed with dil. HCl by boiling for few hours on water bath and subjected to filtration and concentrate the filtrate to yield extract.

Test for Steroids

Libermann & Burchard's test: 2 ml of extract is mixed with chloroform; add 1-2 ml of acetic anhydride and 2 drops of concentrated H_2SO_4 from the sides of the test tube. First red, then blue and finally green colour appears. This is test for steroids.

Salkowski test: To the chloroform extract, few ml of concentrated H_2SO_4 is added. Formation of greenish yellow indicates presence of steroids.

Test for cardiac gylcosides

Keller kiliani test for desoxy sugars (digitoxose, cymarose)

To the concentrated chloroform extract, add few drops of glacial acetic acid, one drop of 5% ferric chloride solution and transfer to test tube containing 2 ml of conc.H_2SO_4. Reddish brown colour appeared at the junction of the two layers and upper layer turns bluish green indicating the presence of desoxy sugar in cardiac glycoside.

Legal's test: Concentrated purified extract dissolved in pyridine and sodium nitroprusside solution was added and make it alkaline. Pink or red colour is produced. Indicates the presence of unsaturated 5 membered lactone ring.

Baljet test: Concentrated purified extract treated with metal picrates of picric acid (sodium picrate). It gives yellow to orange tinge due to unsaturated 5 membered lactone ring.

Test for Anthraquinone Glycosides

Borntrager's test: Petroleum ether (any organic immiscible solvent) extract treated with equal volume of solution of ammonia. Ammonia phase turns to pink or red colour due to derivatives of anthraquinone.

Test for Saponins

1. **Foam test or frothing test:** About 1 ml of extract + 20 ml distilled water → shaken well in graduated cylinder for 15 minutes → 1 cm of persistent foam layer. The frothing indicates the presence of saponins.

2. **Haemolysis test:** To few ml of blood sample add few ml of sample solution. Formation of coagulate indicates the presence of saponins

Test for Flavanoids

1. **Lead acetate test**

   To small quantity of ethanolic extract, add lead acetate solution shows yellow coloured precipitate.

2. **Shinoda's test**

   To the ethanolic extract add 5ml of 95% ethanol and a few drops of concentrated HCl. To this solution 0.5gms of magnesium turnings are added. Observation of pink colouration indicates the presence of flavanoids.

3. **Zn-HCl reduction test:** Heat Sample with zinc and concentrated HCl, the reaction mixture shows the magenta colour.

Volatile oils

1. It have the characteristic odour.
2. The filter paper is not stained permanently with volatile oil.
3. They shows solubility in 90% alcohol.
4. Sample when treated with Sudan III, volatile oil globules stain red or pink colour.